W9-BLY-881

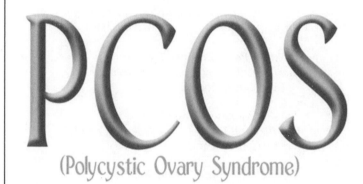

PCOS

(Polycystic Ovary Syndrome)

Hay House Titles of Related Interest

BOOKS

The Body Knows: *How to Tune In to Your Body and Improve Your Health,*
by Caroline M. Sutherland, Medical Intuitive

Doctors Cry, Too: *Essays from the Heart of a Physician,*
by Frank H. Boehm, M.D.

Heal Your Body: *The Mental Causes for Physical Illness and the
Metaphysical Way to Overcome Them,* by Louise L. Hay

Help Me to Heal:
A Practical Guidebook for Patients, Visitors, and Caregivers,
by Bernie S. Siegel, M.D., and Yosaif August

Inner Peace for Busy Women:
Balancing Work, Family, and Your Inner Life,
by Joan Z. Borysenko, Ph.D.

Menopause Made Easy:
How to Make the Right Decisions for the Rest of Your Life,
by Carolle Jean-Murat, M.D.

The Mommy Chronicles:
Sharing the Comedy and Drama of Pregnancy and New Motherhood,
by Sara Ellington and Stephanie Triplett (available March 2005)

CARD DECKS/CALENDAR

Healthy Living Cards: *Ideas for Living Younger Longer,*
by the staff at Canyon Ranch

Self-Care Cards, by Cheryl Richardson

Women's Bodies, Women's Health *Perpetual Flip Calendar,*
by Christiane Northrup, M.D.

Women's Bodies, Women's Wisdom Healing Cards,
by Christiane Northrup, M.D.

All of the above are available at your local bookstore, or may be ordered by visiting:
Hay House USA: **www.hayhouse.com**®; Hay House Australia:
www.hayhouse.com.au; Hay House UK: **www.hayhouse.co.uk;** Hay House South
Africa: **orders@psdprom.co.za** • **www.hayhouse.co.za;**
Hay House India: **www.hayhouse.co.in**

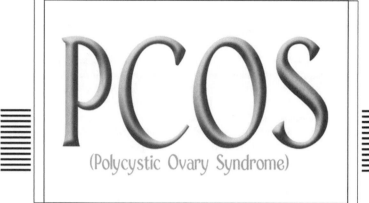
PCOS
(Polycystic Ovary Syndrome)

Your Guide to Self-Care, Emotional
Well-Being, and Medical Support

Colette Harris
with Theresa Cheung

HAY HOUSE, INC.
Carlsbad, California
London • Sydney • Johannesburg
Vancouver • Hong Kong • New Delhi

Copyright © 2004 by Colette Harris

Published and distributed in the United States by: Hay House, Inc.: www.hayhouse.com • *Published and distributed in Australia by:* Hay House Australia Pty. Ltd.: www.hayhouse.com.au • *Published and distributed in the United Kingdom by:* Hay House UK, Ltd.: www.hayhouse.co.uk • *Published and distributed in the Republic of South Africa by:* Hay House SA (Pty), Ltd.: orders@psdprom.co.za • www.hayhouse.co.za • *Distributed in Canada by:* Raincoast: www.raincoast.com • *Published in India by:* Hay House Publishers India: www.hayhouse.co.in

All rights reserved. No part of this book may be reproduced by any mechanical, photographic, or electronic process, or in the form of a phonographic recording; nor may it be stored in a retrieval system, transmitted, or otherwise be copied for public or private use—other than for "fair use" as brief quotations embodied in articles and reviews without prior written permission of the publisher.

The authors of this book do not dispense medical advice or prescribe the use of any technique as a form of treatment for physical or medical problems without the advice of a physician, either directly or indirectly. The intent of the authors is only to offer information of a general nature to help you in your quest for emotional and spiritual well-being. In the event you use any of the information in this book for yourself, which is your constitutional right, the authors and the publisher assume no responsibility for your actions.

Library of Congress Cataloging-in-Publication Data

Harris, Colette.
  PCOS (polycystic ovary syndrome) : your guide to self-care, emotional well-being, and medical support / Colette Harris with Theresa Cheung.
    p. cm.
  Includes bibliographical references.
  ISBN 1-4019-0292-8 (tradepaper)
  1. Polycystic ovary syndrome—Popular works. 2. Infertility—Treatment—Popular works. I. Title: Polycystic ovary syndrome. II. Cheung, Theresa. III. Title.
  RG480.S7H37 2004
  618.1'1—dc22

2004013536

ISBN 13: 978-1-4019-0292-6
ISBN 10: 1-4019-0292-8

10 09 08 07   5 4 3 2
1st printing, September 2004
2nd printing, May 2007

Printed in the United States of America

*For women with PCOS
and the people who support them*

Contents

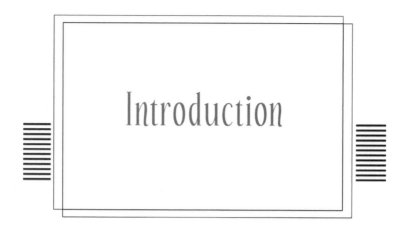

Introduction

You may be reading this book because you have PCOS (poly-cystic ovary syndrome) and have been trying to have a baby, without success, for some time now. Problems with fertility are the number one reason why women visit their doctor and end up being diagnosed with PCOS.

Perhaps you have PCOS and are worried about how the condition may impact your chances of motherhood in the future, or perhaps you're pregnant and worried about being a high-risk pregnancy.

If fertility is a concern for you, you're certainly not alone. Research shows that women with PCOS are more concerned about their fertility than women without, and that this can affect their quality of life.[1]

The first question many women with PCOS ask, even if they don't want a baby right now, is: "Will I be able to have babies when the time is right for me?"

"I've just been diagnosed with PCOS and was told that it means I might not be able to have children! What on earth is this condition? And how can I make sure it doesn't affect me this way?" — Charlotte, 26 years old

"I've got PCOS and the clock is ticking. I haven't met Mr. Right yet, and I sometimes wonder if I ever will. I want to have children, and I'm seriously considering becoming a single mother by choice." — Rachel, 35 years old

"I don't want to have kids right now because I just don't feel ready, but I'm worried that PCOS will affect my future chances of getting pregnant when the time is right for me." — Jenny, 24 years old

If you have PCOS, fertility is a big issue. When your periods are irregular or absent and there are problems with ovulation, you're more likely to have difficulties. Without an egg in the right place at the right time to receive sperm, you can't get pregnant. And even if all this happens, the incidence of miscarriage for women with PCOS is thought to be higher than average.[2]

But don't panic—there *is* some good news. Recent studies show that many women with PCOS get pregnant and give birth to healthy babies once they get some key symptoms under control by balancing underlying hormone levels.

And in many cases, these pregnancies occur without fertility drugs.[3]

"Over 70 percent of women with PCOS do manage to conceive naturally in the end. Over 20 percent manage to conceive with treatment. There is much hope and considerable help for PCOS patients to establish a pregnancy," says renowned expert in reproductive endocrinology, Dr. Samuel Thatcher. "Therapy may be as much as 90 percent effective for fertility problems related to PCOS."

How This Book Works

This book is designed to help you maximize your chances of being able to get pregnant and have a healthy pregnancy. It provides a practical handbook for you to work through as you go on your fertility journey.

1. Chapter 1 explains what PCOS is. Then, at whatever stage of the journey you currently are, the Seven-Step Fertility-Boosting Action Plan in Chapter 2 is a basic set of guidelines for women with PCOS to follow in order to help maximize their ability to conceive.
It will work as a primer for you even if you're not ready to start trying just yet, as a booster if you're trying, and as the foundation for a self-care plan that can be fine-tuned especially for you if you find you need some extra help.

2. That's where Chapter 3 comes in—if you've tried the seven steps and you're still dealing with problems such as irregular periods, then use the scientifically backed information in this section to fine-tune the basic plan by using a proactive approach to self-care and natural therapies that you and your partner can embark on together.

3. Chapters 4 and 5: If you want or need to consider natural or medical fertility treatment, these chapters look at what's available to you as a woman with PCOS. These treatments will work in conjunction with the seven-step plan, which is still your basic self-help guide and will help enhance the effects of any treatment you undertake.

4. Happily, as so many women with PCOS do eventually conceive, Chapter 6 looks at how you can have a healthy pregnancy.

5. All of this can be quite an exhausting process—not only physically, but mentally, too. So Chapters 7 and 8 are full of practical information to help you ride the ups and downs of the PCOS fertility roller coaster, and stay happy and healthy along the way.

Personal PCOS Stories

Because we know that sometimes the best medicine for helping you cope with PCOS is hearing the stories of other women who have the condition and are dealing with it, there are many stories at every stage throughout the book to give you comfort, hope, and inspiration. All the women who are quoted here have PCOS. They've shared their stories with us through support-group meetings we've attended, conversations over dinner with friends, via e-mail groups and chat rooms, and through direct e-mails in response to requests we've made at the end of lectures or flyers in PCOS support-group newsletters and meetings. And so that you know where we're coming from, here are our own PCOS fertility stories to kick things off.

Colette's Story

"Don't worry, there's a lot they can do nowadays for women who can't have children," said the ultrasound technician who was scanning me at the appointment I'd fought for months to get.

"What do you mean?" I asked.

"You've got polycystic ovary syndrome," he said.

"What do you mean?" I repeated blankly.

"I think you'd better ask your doctor about that," was the reply.

It was December 1996. I was 23 years old, and after months of failing health after coming off the Pill—from hair loss to acne, loss of my periods to gaining almost 30 pounds, fatigue so overwhelming that the thought of climbing a flight of stairs made me cry, and mood swings like Jekyll and Hyde—I finally had a diagnosis. I was infertile. And suddenly, for the first time in my life, I began to think that I wanted children, even though deep down I knew it wasn't the right time.

I'd spent months trying to convince my doctors that there was something wrong with me beyond their sense of "Who doesn't feel tired these days?" And here I was, after my doctor sent me for blood tests and an ultrasound scan but refused to tell me why, being told that I couldn't have children and I had polycystic ovary syndrome.

I went back to the doctor clutching my results.

"Congratulations," he said. I looked at him in confusion.

"Well, you're pregnant, I take it?" he said, nodding at the print of the scan in my hand.

"Well, actually, I've just found out I can't have children," I said. To give him credit, he was quite embarrassed.

Even though we hadn't gotten off to the best start, at least he admitted that he didn't know anything about PCOS and was happy to refer me to a gynecologist who he thought might help (the earliest appointment was five months later). But he did reassure me that if I went on the Pill to get rid of the symptoms, I could come back when I wanted kids, and they'd do their best to treat me with the miracles of modern medicine. "There's no reason why you shouldn't be able to have children if you want them," the doctor told me.

Although I was confused, being told one minute I was infertile, and the next that I probably wasn't, my anxiety about whether I wanted to become a mom had been put on hold by my doctor's reassurance that there would be options for me if I chose to go down that route. Not only had I never envisioned myself as a mother, having very mixed feelings about even wanting to have kids at all, but I was also in a great new relationship (which I'm happily still in now, seven years later!), which was already reeling under the stresses and strains of my hideous PCOS symptoms. Why on earth would I want to bring the "baby or not" question into that mix, either for myself or my partner? It was enough to come to terms with getting a mustache, with bursting into tears at the slightest sappy moment on TV, or with having breasts so tender and swollen that I had to sleep on my back.

Dealing with those symptoms was uppermost in my mind when I decided to not just wait for another five months in misery while I inched up the gynecologist's waiting list. Instead, I'd turn PCOS detective and see what steps I could take myself to deal with the condition. I read everything I could find (not much in 1997—the Internet sites that are now available, thank goodness, just weren't around then), and talked to doctors, medical herbalists, nutritionists, pharmacists, and other women with PCOS, whom I'd been lucky enough to meet through the fledgling UK charity for women with PCOS, Verity. And I began to realize that what I ate, how stressed I was, how much exercise I did, and how much toxic input went into my mind and body could all be having a massive effect on my hormonal balance and insulin resistance.

I made myself a test case and tried a natural and healthy eating plan, acupuncture, medical herbalism, and nutritional supplements, and I was astounded by the results: My periods came back within six weeks, the weight started coming off, my painful lumpy spots were reduced massively, my hair loss stopped, and my moods evened out.

The gynecologist said I seemed to know more about the condition than she did. "Whatever you're doing is working really well," she remarked. "I'd suggest you carry on."

So I did—and I've kept it up all this time.

But now that I'm nearly 31, many of my friends are having kids and asking me when I'm going to, and those words from my ultrasound scan have been coming back to haunt me. Before I started researching this book, I knew that any woman's fertility starts to decline after 35, and that's there's a lot medical science can offer women with PCOS if they have problems getting pregnant. But now I also know that 70 percent of women with PCOS actually end up getting pregnant naturally, that fertility treatment is thought to be around 90 percent successful for women with PCOS, and that there's a massive amount you can do with your own diet and lifestyle to boost your fertility and the success of *any* fertility treatment you have. So although I haven't made my choices about motherhood yet, I'm delighted to feel that I *have* choices, and that I can take an active role in managing my own fertility.

Writing this book has been a fascinating journey. I've felt reassured that I'm a woman who happens to have PCOS, not just a PCOS patient. I'm a woman who has to decide, like any woman, whether motherhood is something I want, and I'm determined not to let my PCOS panic me into making a hasty decision.

There's no doubt that having PCOS brings your fertility into sharp focus. But writing this book has helped me see it more clearly than ever: Having PCOS doesn't mean you can't experience motherhood. In fact, your chances of success are higher than ever now, with more and more research being done (lots of which you'll find in this book), and as it becomes more obvious that your diet, stress levels, and lifestyle can all have a hugely positive impact. I wish I could find that ultrasound technician and tell him to pass on the good news to anyone else he scans for PCOS!

So if you're at the same stage as I am, or your heart is telling you that it's time to have a baby, or you're already trying, or you're looking to address problems or face emotional losses and work out how to move forward, I sincerely hope that this book brings you some information, comfort, inspiration, and practical ideas that will help you on your own fertility journey.

Theresa's Story

I used to be an energetic person, but everything changed a few months after I stopped taking the Pill. I felt as if I were falling apart. I became anxious and moody, and it was difficult to concentrate. I was depressed one moment, agitated the next, and perpetually tired. Some days even walking up the stairs was exhausting.

After several months of feeling terrible, I went to see my doctor. He examined me and assured me I wasn't dying, then asked me when I'd had my last period. I told him I hadn't had one since I stopped taking the Pill about eight months ago. He told me that I had amenorrhea. I'd never heard of the word and discovered that it is the medical term used to describe a lack of menstruation in women before menopause. I didn't know what to think. Was I going into menopause early?

The doctor explained that many women experience amenorrhea at some point in their lives, especially when they're under stress or after they come off the Pill. He asked me if I'd been working too hard, then he told me to relax—it would sort itself out by the time I was to come back in six months. He even joked, saying that I should enjoy the freedom of not having a monthly cycle. He also suggested going back on the Pill, but I told him I didn't want to. I'd only had a few irregular periods before going on birth control in my late teens, and I wanted to see if I could menstruate naturally.

My husband assured me that everything would be all right. I appreciated his support, but how could he understand what it felt like to be a woman without her natural rhythms? Having just gotten married, I never knew what to say when friends kept asking when, or if, we were going to start a family. I didn't even have the choice.

When I returned in six months to see my doctor, my periods were still absent, my skin was breaking out, and my hair lacked shine. I looked and felt much older than 28. I exercised and watched my diet, but it was getting harder and harder to keep motivated. My husband was worried, since he'd never seen me so depressed, and the weight was piling on.

This time it was recommended that I get an ultrasound. I was told that there was a slight problem with my ovaries, but my doctor said that it was just one of those things, and if I didn't want to start a family right now, then there was little point in offering me treatment. Once again, he suggested the Pill; once again, I refused.

I never had time to think things through, as my husband and I were due to leave for the United States for a three-year assignment. It was a very exciting time, and my health took a backseat while I adjusted to a new way of life. I kept hoping that my periods would return, but they never did.

A year or so after we'd settled in the U.S., I finally visited a gynecologist. When I explained that I didn't have periods, I was given progesterone to induce one and told to wait and see if my body could regulate itself so that my periods would start again. They didn't. By now I was 32 and really starting to think about babies. Even though I'd planned on having children in my mid- to late 30s, I could see that time wasn't on my side. Obviously something was wrong.

I was referred to a specialist for a series of tests. The specialist said that I had an excess amount of male hormone circulating in my body, which was interfering with my reproductive cycle, and it was likely I had cysts on my ovaries. An examination confirmed this. I was told that I had polycystic ovaries, and as long as I had this condition, it could be difficult for me to get pregnant. I was told that the condition was very common, which I suppose was meant to make me feel better, but it didn't really. I heard the word *cyst* and imagined the worst. All I thought was, *If the condition is so common, why haven't I heard of it? Does this mean I can't have babies?*

Despite feeling anxious, it was a huge relief to finally find out what was wrong and to be taken seriously. Without really knowing what was going on, I agreed to have hormonal treatments: progesterone to encourage a period, the fertility drug Clomid to induce ovulation, and hormone injections to release the egg if it was ready. It was an emotional roller coaster of a month, when each day seemed the longest ever. The treatment was all I could think about. It was painful and difficult, as I'd never wanted to have kids as much as I did now. It wasn't easy for my husband, either—I'll never forget the look on his face when I'd had my injection, and it was suggested that we have intercourse that evening, the following morning, afternoon, and evening, and then again the day after. No pressure on the poor guy!

I jumped for joy when the pregnancy test turned positive after my first attempt. Nine months later, I gave birth to a beautiful baby boy. But within a year I was panicking again: I'd always planned on two children, and my periods hadn't returned. We had now returned to the U.K., so I visited my doctor again. I was more hopeful this time, as I knew what was wrong with me. I told him I had PCOS and gave him my medical reports from the U.S. I couldn't believe it when he refused to even look at them and wanted my husband and me to go in for basic fertility testing. I didn't want to put either of us through all that again. I decided to change doctors, and thankfully found one who knew about PCOS and was willing to listen. I had the same treatment as before, and this time got pregnant after the third attempt. Nine months later, I had a beautiful baby girl.

Now that my family was complete, I really turned my attention to my PCOS. A year after my baby girl was born, I still wasn't menstruating. I visited three more doctors, all of whom suggested the Pill, but this wasn't what I wanted. I wanted a natural approach. I did lots of my own research, talked to experts, and even wrote a series of articles and a book about hormonal imbalance in women. Then I had a stroke of luck. My editor suggested that I get together with fellow PCOS sufferer Colette Harris, who had already written a groundbreaking and best-selling book on the subject. Colette needed a writer to work with her on *The PCOS Diet Book*—a book designed to encourage women with PCOS to treat their condition through diet, supplements, exercise, and stress relief. This was almost too good to be true. I could write, learn about, and treat my condition at the same time.

Over an 18-month period, the natural approach has worked brilliantly. My periods have returned naturally and have been as regular as clockwork ever since. I've also got my weight under control, and my skin and hair look healthy again. Unless we decide to try for another baby, I have no way of knowing if my do-it-yourself techniques would have resulted in pregnancy, but I do know that I've never felt healthier and happier. The regularity of my periods indicates a healthy and fertile reproductive cycle. I also think about how far I've come in the past five years. Back then, I had no idea what was wrong with me and was convinced I'd never have a family of my own. I hope that my experience will give hope and inspiration to every woman diagnosed with PCOS who's concerned about her fertility.

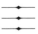

Chapter One

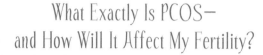

What Exactly Is PCOS— and How Will It Affect My Fertility?

The key to understanding how and why PCOS can affect your fertility is to come to grips with what it is. Unfortunately, it's quite a complicated answer, but the basics are that polycystic ovary syndrome (PCOS) is a metabolic disorder that can cause hormonal imbalances and a whole array of symptoms, including irregular or absent periods, problems with fertility, acne, hair loss, weight gain, excess facial hair, diabetes, high blood pressure, fatigue, and mood swings. These conditions can all be mild or severe, and yours may not be the same as another women with PCOS—there are so many symptoms that you can end up with a combination that's very specific to you, even if the underlying cause in PCOS cases is the same.

If you've got PCOS, you're certainly not alone. Around 10 percent of women have polycystic ovaries, even though many of them may not know it—they may have been misdiagnosed with PMS or stress, for instance; or they may have PCO, which means they have polycystic ovaries on an ultrasound scan but not any outward signs of them.[4] (When a woman is symptom free, the polycystic ovaries show that she has a built-in predisposition to developing PCOS. If she puts on weight or comes under a great deal of stress, she many develop the problems listed above.)

The Role of Sex Hormones

Often, the imbalance in the sex hormones that are responsible for symptoms such as excess hair or acne is also interfering with your ability to ovulate. You can usually tell if you're not ovulating properly by whether or not you're having regular periods, as a "normal" menstrual cycle involves ovulation followed by a period.

The Normal Menstrual Cycle

In a normal menstrual cycle, the first half, called the *follicular phase*, starts on the first day of your period and lasts for about 14 days. In this phase, the pituitary gland releases low levels of FSH (the follicle-stimulating hormone) to stimulate the follicles in the ovary to ripen their eggs and produce the hormone estrogen, which causes the lining of the womb to start to thicken in preparation for pregnancy. When levels of estrogen are high enough, the pituitary gland produces a large amount of LH (luteinizing hormone), and the dominant matured follicle in the ovary releases its egg into the fallopian tubes toward the womb in a process called *ovulation*.

After ovulation comes the second stage of the menstrual cycle, called the *luteal phase*. Here, the cells from the burst follicle collapse to form a cyst called the *corpus luteum*. The corpus luteum now produces progesterone as the main hormone of the second half of the cycle. Progesterone causes the thickened lining of the womb to secrete nutrients ready to receive the fertilized egg. If the egg is fertilized, it will implant itself in the womb, and the corpus luteum will continue to produce progesterone to protect the pregnancy. If it isn't fertilized 14 days after ovulation, the corpus luteum stops producing progesterone and estrogen. The thickened womb lining starts to break down and is shed as a period, ready for the whole cycle to start again.

If you've got PCOS, there's often a problem with the hormones that trigger ovulation every month, which means that not only are irregular or absent periods highly likely, but getting pregnant can be more difficult. On top of that, when ovulation isn't successful, you don't get the surge of progesterone to balance the estrogen in the second half of your cycle, which is normally the way things happen—instead, your estrogen levels stay the same and can cause symptoms such as bloating, fatigue, absent or irregular periods, hot flashes, and dizziness, as well as mood swings and depression.

The Role of Insulin

If you have PCOS, it's not only your sex hormones that are out of balance and causing an ovulation disturbance. Your body's hormonal system, known as the *endocrine system,* is a web of interconnections, so an imbalance in one hormone can affect the balance of others, too. And in PCOS, insulin is a key hormone that can add to the problem. This is because many women with PCOS are insulin resistant, a condition that makes weight gain easy and weight loss hard—and we know that being overweight can also interfere with your body's ability to ovulate.

Insulin is the hormone that helps cells absorb sugar from the bloodstream. So after a meal, when the blood-sugar levels are high and the body wants to store some for energy to use later, the pancreas has to make extra insulin to get the body to store that sugar. The high surge in insulin means that the body goes into sugar-storage overdrive and practically clears the bloodstream of any sugar, leading to low blood-sugar levels and cravings for more sugary food. This becomes a vicious cycle that can lead to putting on even more weight. If this goes on for years, it can wear out the pancreas's ability to make any more insulin and increase the risk of diabetes.

What Are the "Cysts"?

High insulin levels also somehow increase the body's output of the sex hormone testosterone, which can cause excess body hair and acne and affect the ovary's ability to mature and release an egg every month.

Even though there's usually enough follicle-stimulating hormone (FSH) to encourage your egg follicles to develop, there isn't the right balance of other hormones, such as progesterone or luteinizing hormone (LH), to encourage the egg inside it to mature. And those empty follicles that don't release an egg are the "cysts" you may have seen on your ultrasound when you were diagnosed.[5]

(These cysts are thought to be follicles that have failed to develop completely in order to release an egg. They're not the same as ovarian cysts, which are normally bigger and found within the ovary.)

These cysts, then, are just another symptom of the hormonal imbalances you get when you have PCOS. They're not the cause—and it's interesting to note that in many women who get their diet and lifestyle back on track, or use medication to help deal with their PCOS, the "cysts" often decrease in size and number in the same way that any other symptom, such as acne, might.

So, PCOS is a metabolic disorder that triggers a series of hormonal imbalances, including raised testosterone, lack of LH, and potential insulin resistance, all of which can have an effect on your body's ability to ovulate regularly.

And this is how PCOS, and not the "cysts" on your ovaries, can affect fertility.

What's the Difference Between PCOS, Syndrome X, and Syndrome O?

You may have also heard this group of symptoms described as *Syndrome X* and *Syndrome O*. *Syndrome X* is a term coined by a group of researchers at Stanford University to describe a cluster of symptoms, that, when occurring together, increase a person's risk of diabetes, hypertension, and heart disease. These symptoms are high blood pressure, insulin resistance, low levels of good cholesterol (HDL), and obesity.

Syndrome O is a term used by reproductive endocrinologist Dr. Ronald Feinberg to describe a condition of insulin overproduction and ovarian disruption that can lead to abnormal bleeding, missed menses, and fertility problems.

Feinberg suggests that Syndrome O should replace the term *PCOS*, as many women with PCOS don't have any significant cysts when checked by ultrasound, although there is still evidence that they may be at risk of developing insulin resistance. He also believes that Syndrome O is easier to teach; most women with PCOS who were polled by the Polycystic Ovarian Syndrome Association (PCOSA) desired a name change for the syndrome, recognizing that it's a whole-body female problem, not just an ovarian disorder.

Feinberg has a point, but on the face of it, there really isn't much to distinguish his definition of Syndrome O and the standard definition of PCO and PCOS. It's really just a new name for the cluster of symptoms we recognize as PCOS.

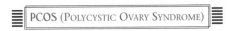

How Will PCOS Affect My Fertility?

However, these symptoms don't mean you're infertile. Infertility means being unable to have a baby when you want one, and as we've seen, 70 percent of women with PCOS conceive naturally. If you've got PCOS and have absent or irregular periods, or problems with ovulation, you're not infertile—you have a condition known as *subfertility*. This means that getting pregnant may not be as simple for you as it is for some women, but it's by no means an impossible feat. And it's amazing how much you can do yourself to boost your chances of success.

This is where self-help comes in. A sperm can be a champion swimmer, but if ovulation doesn't happen and there's no egg to fertilize, there will be no pregnancy. But in PCOS, there are often lots of potential eggs there, just waiting to mature. As the hormonal imbalance of PCOS is the cause of problems with fertility, if you can bring your hormones back into a more regular pattern, you can increase your chances of triggering ovulation. And that's what the information in the fertility-boosting plan in this book is designed to help you do.

How Will PCOS Affect Pregnancy?

The right hormonal conditions are also essential for a healthy full-term pregnancy—which is why miscarriage is associated with PCOS. If you know what you're looking out for, you can, in partnership with your health-care practitioner, take an active role.

Many of the factors that can upset hormonal balance and hinder fertility or cause miscarriage are within your power to control or change. Simple changes in your diet, lifestyle, and attitude can make all the difference. For instance, research suggests that what you eat is very significant for your fertility.[6] Understanding nutrition and correctly supplementing your diet is the first essential step to balancing hormones naturally. Countless studies also show that stress can affect fertility and upset hormonal balance, so managing your stress levels will also help.[7] Weight-management problems can also hinder pregnancy. "What I try to show my patients with PCOS," says Dr. Robert Franklin, clinical professor of obstetrics and gynecology at Baylor College of Medicine in Houston, Texas, "is how her excess or under-weight affects her hormones and her ability to get pregnant." So, tackling any weight issues will also boost your chances.

That isn't to say that you'll necessarily get pregnant overnight if you eat well, de-stress, and deal with weight problems. After all, even "normal" couples are expected to try for a year before undergoing any medical investigation, and there are other factors you need to bear in mind that may be causing problems with fertility. For example, researchers believe that sperm counts have been reduced by more than 40 percent in the last 50 years, with environmental pollutants from plastics and toxins, such as pesticides, thought to inhibit fertility due to their ability to act like estrogen and disturb hormonal balance.[8] Factors like these show that far from being something you have little control over, there's a lot you can do to boost your fertility.

Why Does It Happen?

No one is really sure why women with PCOS can't produce the correct balance of hormones so that an ovary can develop and release an egg. There are several theories, including those that suggest that inappropriate levels of the hormones testosterone, insulin, cortisol, and LH are the culprits, but the general consensus is that PCOS is most likely a disorder that runs in families.[9] So if your mother had PCOS and irregular periods, chances are that you will, too. Factors such as diet, lifestyle, weight, and pollution also contribute to the development and severity of your symptoms, and although you can't change your genetic heritage, you *can* change your diet and lifestyle. You can start to be the driver of your hormonal life to maximize your chances of health and fertility.

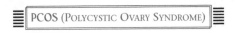
Use this book as a practical tool to help boost your fertility levels so that your body and mind are in as good a shape as possible for when you do decide to try to have a baby, or to help you if you're already trying now. And if you're having further problems, the self-help steps throughout the book will also help you get the most from any fertility treatments you may decide to have.

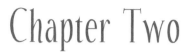

Chapter Two

Your Seven-Step
Fertility-Boosting Action Plan

Getting pregnant isn't just about having sex. Research shows that everything you do in the three or four months *before* trying to conceive can be as important as the sex itself.[a]

What you drink, eat, or breathe; the work you do; how stressed you are; how you feel about yourself—everything matters. Any one of these factors can mean the difference between conceiving and having a healthy baby and not conceiving, especially if you're taking longer to get pregnant than you thought you would.

There's a lot you can do to prepare your body for a healthy pregnancy, and that's what this section of the book is all about. It's an action plan specifically designed for women with PCOS to boost their fertility.

The good news is that the great majority of these things are under your control. The even better news is that this self-help approach has helped countless women with PCOS get pregnant and have healthy babies.

How to Use the Plan

This PCOS fertility-boosting plan is designed to get you into the best possible shape, both mentally and physically, in order to maximize your chances of conceiving and having a healthy baby. This plan is your basic foundation—you may need nothing more than these seven steps to bring about pregnancy. However, if you're having problems, these steps will help your body and mind cope better with overcoming them. And if you're having fertility treatments of any kind, the seven steps will enhance the effectiveness of those treatments, as well as your ability to cope with the treatments both physically and emotionally.

In an ideal world, we'd recommend that you follow this plan for three to four months before you try to conceive or turn to assisted conception. This is because the healthier you are before you get pregnant or start fertility treatment, the better your chances of conceiving, and of the pregnancy resulting in a healthy baby.

World-renowned fertility expert Dr. Niels Lauersen states: "While it was once believed that obstetrical treatment should begin only after a conception is confirmed, today most forward-thinking physicians recognize that many problems can be prevented when the same care begins before you get pregnant." This concept is known as *preconceptual care,* a program of healthy living for you and your partner, which will boost your chances of fertility.

The Importance of Preconceptual Care

Many fertility specialists now recommend preconception care whenever a couple decides they want to start a family, and this has particular benefits for women with PCOS. Research on PCOS sufferers has shown how effective diet and lifestyle changes can be for the condition, and how it can not only improve symptoms such as irregular periods, weight gain, acne, and facial hair, but can also dramatically increase the chances of both conception and a healthy, full-term pregnancy.[10-13]

Whether you're about to try to have a baby for the first time, or are at the stage where you're considering fertility drugs, the action plan is a good idea. Not only might you get a surprise natural pregnancy (the National Institute of Environmental Health Sciences in North Carolina showed that couples who failed to conceive naturally within the first year did conceive naturally in the second year[b]), but you will also enhance the power of the fertility treatment itself. "After alteration in lifestyle," says PCOS expert Dr. Samuel Thatcher, "some women with PCOS can avoid ever being seen in a fertility clinic."

Your Four-Month Preconception Plan

Even when your future baby is still a longing or a twinkle in your eye, you and your partner can both be taking steps toward a healthy conception. The healthier you both are, the better your chances of conceiving sooner rather than later, and of the pregnancy producing a healthy baby at the end.

Now, three to four months is the recommended period of time for preconceptual care because it takes about three months for a new batch of sperm to be made, and three months for a woman's egg to develop from its follicle and be released. It also takes between six weeks and three months to eliminate certain toxins from your system properly, and to raise the level of crucial fertility-boosting nutrients in your blood serum. Research spearheaded by Foresight and backed up by U.K. doctors suggests that a good three- to four-month program of healthy living will maximize your chances of conception, whether you want to try now or in the future.[14]

Taking care of yourself before you get pregnant is not only important for your fertility—it's crucial for your baby-to-be, too. The egg that's released at conception is the product of your diet and lifestyle, and experts now believe that what a woman eats prior to conception is just as significant to the health of the baby as what she eats during pregnancy.[15]

According to Irwin Emanuel, M.D., professor of epidemiology and pediatrics at the University of Washington in Seattle, "If you are undernourished, your baby could well become 'programmed' at conception to develop high blood pressure, clotting disorders, abnormal glucose, insulin and cholesterol problems, and even hormonal problems like PCOS."

The first weeks of pregnancy are increasingly understood to be the most important in terms of fetal development, as that's when all the major organs—heart, lungs, liver, kidneys, nervous system—are formed. Remember, women are already two weeks pregnant before they miss a period, so eating well in the time leading up to a pregnancy is really important.

Your Seven Steps to Fertility

Every woman with PCOS is unique, and there's not one magic formula that will work for all. But making healthy diet and lifestyle choices before you get pregnant can yield dramatic results. For at least three months before trying to conceive, you (and your partner) should:

1. Manage your weight.

2. Get as fit and as well as you can.

3. Reduce the level of stress in your life.

4. Eat fresh, healthy food, and make sure that you get your pro-fertility nutrients.

5. Detox your diet and your lifestyle to get rid of anti-fertility chemicals.

6. Ask yourself if you're ready.

7. Enjoy your sex life.

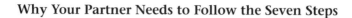

Why Your Partner Needs to Follow the Seven Steps

A good preconceptual-care program involves getting both partners into the best possible physical and mental shape before trying to have a baby. In couples with fertility problems, it's thought that approximately one third can be attributed to the male partner, one third to the female partner, and one third to a combination of both partners. For couples who are having difficulty getting pregnant, doing all seven steps to fertility together is important because although your baby will be nourished inside you, it takes both your egg and your partner's sperm to make a baby.

If both partners are physically and emotionally fit, then the healthier your eggs and sperm are, and the better your chances of getting and staying pregnant will be. Never lose sight of the fact that getting pregnant takes two, and there may be other problems aside from PCOS. If you're not as fertile as you could be due to irregular ovulation, and your partner has a lower than normal sperm count, this can reduce your chances even further.

For men, the most common problem is not just how many sperm there are, but also sperm quality. In other words, are they strong and fit enough to reach and penetrate a ripe egg? Both sperm quality and quantity can be affected by lifestyle factors such as poor diet, stress, too little exercise, smoking, and alcohol. In addition, your partner should avoid hot baths, tight underwear, exposure to heat, traffic fumes, and long hours sitting and driving. Why? Because studies have shown that all these factors can have a negative effect on sperm quality and quantity.[16] This gives a man a great deal of control over his own fertility, and numerous studies have shown that simple diet and lifestyle changes can improve sperm in as little as three months.[17]

Step One: Manage Your Weight

> *"About a year ago I was diagnosed with PCOS and told that if I wanted to start a family it might be harder than I thought.*

I was told that I'd improve my chances if I lost some weight. It was a shock, and at first I felt completely overwhelmed. Steve and I had been trying for a baby for a while now, and this wasn't good news. As for losing weight, I'd been trying for years and had tried every diet in the book, so how was I going to manage it now?

"My doctor referred me to a dietitian who had treated women with PCOS before. I was given advice about healthy food choices and was encouraged to take up some gentle exercise—so I started walking to work instead of taking the bus. Within four months, I'd gone down two dress sizes, my periods got regular, and my acne improved. I felt wonderful for the first time in years.

"Then about a year after being diagnosed, when I was just about to go back to my doctor for fertility treatment something amazing happened: I got pregnant." — Charlotte, 33 years old

Your Ideal Body Weight

Carrying too much body fat can make symptoms of PCOS (including irregular periods) worse, and can stop you from getting pregnant. Losing weight, if you have weight to lose, can improve symptoms and boost your fertility. So if you have PCOS and are concerned about fertility, being around the right weight for your height could prove crucial. Your ideal weight for health and fertility is determined by your body mass index, or BMI. A BMI between 21 and 25 is perfect, and between 23 and 24 is ideal for conception. For the average woman, 27 percent of her weight consists of body fat.

Body Mass Index Table

	Normal						Overweight					Obese										Extreme Obesity														
BMI	19	20	21	22	23	24	25	26	27	28	29	30	31	32	33	34	35	36	37	38	39	40	41	42	43	44	45	46	47	48	49	50	51	52	53	54
Height (inches)												\newline Body Weight (pounds)																								
58	91	96	100	105	110	115	119	124	129	134	138	143	148	153	158	162	167	172	177	181	186	191	196	201	205	210	215	220	224	229	234	239	244	248	253	258
59	94	99	104	109	114	119	124	128	133	138	143	148	153	158	163	168	173	178	183	188	193	198	203	208	212	217	222	227	232	237	242	247	252	257	262	267
60	97	102	107	112	118	123	128	133	138	143	148	153	158	163	168	174	179	184	189	194	199	204	209	215	220	225	230	235	240	245	250	255	261	266	271	276
61	100	106	111	116	122	127	132	137	143	148	153	158	164	169	174	180	185	190	195	201	206	211	217	222	227	232	238	243	248	254	259	264	269	275	280	285
62	104	109	115	120	126	131	136	142	147	153	158	164	169	175	180	186	191	196	202	207	213	218	224	229	235	240	246	251	256	262	267	273	278	284	289	295
63	107	113	118	124	130	135	141	146	152	158	163	169	175	180	186	191	197	203	208	214	220	225	231	237	242	248	254	259	265	270	278	282	287	293	299	304
64	110	116	122	128	134	140	145	151	157	163	169	174	180	186	192	197	204	209	215	221	227	232	238	244	250	256	262	267	273	279	285	291	296	302	308	314
65	114	120	126	132	138	144	150	156	162	168	174	180	186	192	198	204	210	216	222	228	234	240	246	252	258	264	270	276	282	288	294	300	306	312	318	324
66	118	124	130	136	142	148	155	161	167	173	179	186	192	198	204	210	216	223	229	235	241	247	253	260	266	272	278	284	291	297	303	309	315	322	328	334
67	121	127	134	140	146	153	159	166	172	178	185	191	198	204	211	217	223	230	236	242	249	255	261	268	274	280	287	293	299	306	312	319	325	331	338	344
68	125	131	138	144	151	158	164	171	177	184	190	197	203	210	216	223	230	236	243	249	256	262	269	276	282	289	295	302	308	315	322	328	335	341	348	354
69	128	135	142	149	155	162	169	176	182	189	196	203	209	216	223	230	236	243	250	257	263	270	277	284	291	297	304	311	318	324	331	338	345	351	358	365
70	132	139	146	153	160	167	174	181	188	195	202	209	216	222	229	236	243	250	257	264	271	278	285	292	299	306	313	320	327	334	341	348	355	362	369	376
71	136	143	150	157	165	172	179	186	193	200	208	215	222	229	236	243	250	257	265	272	279	286	293	301	308	315	322	329	338	343	351	358	365	372	379	386
72	140	147	154	162	169	177	184	191	199	206	213	221	228	235	242	250	258	265	272	279	287	294	302	309	316	324	331	338	346	353	361	368	375	383	390	397
73	144	151	159	166	174	182	189	197	204	212	219	227	235	242	250	257	265	272	280	288	295	302	310	318	325	333	340	348	355	363	371	378	386	393	401	408
74	148	155	163	171	179	186	194	202	210	218	225	233	241	249	256	264	272	280	287	295	303	311	319	326	334	342	350	358	365	373	381	389	396	404	412	420
75	152	160	168	176	184	192	200	208	216	224	232	240	248	256	264	272	279	287	295	303	311	319	327	335	343	351	359	367	375	383	391	399	407	415	423	431
76	156	164	172	180	189	197	205	213	221	230	238	246	254	263	271	279	287	295	304	312	320	328	336	344	353	361	369	377	385	394	402	410	418	426	435	443

Source: Adapted from *Clinical Guidelines on the Identification, Evaluation, and Treatment of Overweight and Obesity in Adults: The Evidence Report.*

Why Weight Is Important for Fertility

A certain amount of body fat is vital to maintain your menstrual cycle, and it's essential to fertility, since women need body fat in order to ovulate. In fact, young girls don't begin their periods until they have at least 17 percent body fat. Studies have shown that 50 percent of women who have a BMI (Body Mass Index) below 20.7 are infertile.[18]

If your BMI is lower than 20, you may want to delay trying to have a baby until you adjust your diet to give your body the resources it needs. Low body weight and sudden weight loss due to a poor diet can disrupt hormonal balance and stop you from ovulating—think of it as nature's way of preventing conception when Mom isn't properly nourished. Having said that, women who are underweight or eating poorly do conceive, but they face a higher risk of miscarriage or giving birth to a baby who is underweight or premature. Infants with low birth weight are vulnerable to infection and prone to feeding problems in the early weeks of life.

However, you can have too much of a good thing. The 2002 figures from the U.K.'s Office for National Statistics show that more than half of all British women are either overweight or clinically obese, having a BMI over 30. Being overweight can interfere with ovulation because the extra fat produces excess estrogen in your system, causing an imbalance in the ratio of the reproductive hormones needed for egg ripening and release.

If your BMI is outside the fertile range, we recommend that you delay trying to get pregnant until you find ways to manage the situation (see our PCOS Weight-Loss and Gain Tips on the following pages). We don't recommend dieting, because doing so can mean that you aren't giving your body the nutrients it needs to ovulate regularly and stay healthy.

We know that both PCOS and obesity increase the risk of infertility, but thankfully the effect is quickly reversed.[19–21] Even losing a small amount of weight can be enough to stimulate ovulation again and make periods regular.[22] A study by the University of Adelaide in 1995 involved 12 overweight women who weren't ovulating.[23–4]

After following a six-month program of diet and exercise, 11 of them conceived naturally. Another study by the University of Milan in 2003 involved 33 overweight women with PCOS who lost 5 percent of their body weight.[25] Ten pregnancies occurred, 15 women experienced spontaneous ovulation, and 18 had a resumption of regular cycles.

If you've got PCOS and think you're overweight, don't panic! Your ideal weight for fertility is probably heavier than you think. The ideal body weight for a woman's fertility covers a wide range, but if you're at the low or high end of the range, it can increase the chances of irregular periods without ovulation. This is a known as *anovulation*—and when no egg is released, you can't get pregnant.

How Weight Affects PCOS Symptoms

Research shows that not only are women with PCOS more likely to be overweight, but being overweight makes symptoms of PCOS worse, especially fertility problems.[23,26-7] If you have PCOS, in addition to your body's typical reaction to restricted food intake (that is, your body goes into starvation mode and your metabolism—the rate at which your body uses the calories or energy from food—slows down so much that you reach a point where even though you're eating less, you can't lose weight), you have another hurdle to face. It's been shown that women with PCOS actually store fat more efficiently and burn calories more slowly than women who don't have the condition.[28] You're in a catch-22 situation. Your inability to lose weight can lead to comfort eating, so you end up feeling trapped in a vicious cycle, with the pounds piling on.

But don't lose heart—even with PCOS, you can regain control of the situation. For women with this syndrome, the best way to lose weight isn't to diet, but simply to eat healthfully and increase your amount of exercise. This helps you control your blood sugar levels to reduce cravings for sugary foods, as well as helping you burn off more calories. "Of utmost important to a patient with PCOS who has weight to lose," says Dr. Robert Franklin, professor of obstetrics and gynecology at Baylor College of Medicine in

Houston, Texas, "is her realization that fast or fad diets will not help—she must follow a diet and exercise program that she can live with for the rest of her life."

Your PCOS Weight-Loss Guidelines

- The basic rule is to burn off more calories than you take in, so you need to exercise regularly!

- Aim for a slow, gradual weight loss of no more than two pounds a week. (It may not sound like much, but it soon adds up.) Aim to get into your ideal weight range, not reach the bottom of it.

- Include more fresh fruits and vegetables in your diet. Remember that a glass of diluted fresh-squeezed juice and a plate of frozen vegetables count, too.

- Eat healthy, fresh, preferably organic food—it only takes ten minutes to whip up some stir fry, a bowl of crunchy salad, or some homemade soup.

- Get into the habit of snacking on healthful foods throughout the day to keep your blood-sugar levels on an even keel. Start your day with a good breakfast, have a healthy mid-morning snack (such as an apple and a couple of almonds), a nutritious lunch, a mid-afternoon snack (such as carrot sticks with a low-fat cheese dip), and a light supper.

- Don't eat big meals after 8 P.M.

- Limit your consumption of animal and dairy fats. Only eat lean, grilled meats and low-fat dairy products.

- Try to drink at least six to eight glasses of fresh water a day.

- Limit your intake of sugar, candies, cakes, cookies, salt, alcohol, caffeine, and foods high in chemicals, additives, and preservatives, such as many ready-made meals or canned produce.

- Increase your intake of fiber by eating more fruits and vegetables and cereals such as muesli, and by choosing brown rice, bread, and pasta.

- Eat good-quality protein (lean meats, nonfat dairy products, nuts, and seeds) with every meal.

- Aim to eat fish at least twice a week, and nuts and seeds (flax, sunflower, hemp, walnuts, cashews) daily.

- Watch your portion size. If you have PCOS, your body stores more calories from the food you do eat, and it's amazing how much less your body needs than your appetite wants.

- Chew thoroughly, and put your knife and fork down between each mouthful—taking your time means you'll feel fuller more quickly.

- Remember the 80/20 rule: Doing well 80 percent of the time is enough and gives you the room for treats and a night off 20 percent of the time. You can't always eat healthfully, and the occasional treat—a bar of chocolate or bag of chips—doesn't mean that you've failed. It's the excesses that are dangerous. It's important that you enjoy your food and allow your-self the occasional indulgence, so no food is off-limits.

- Do more exercise so that you can eat plenty of nutri-tious food but still lose weight—it can be a brisk 20-minute walk every day to start with, as long as you start doing more than you're doing now. Exercise is really key if you have PCOS, so you need to *get* moti-vated and *stay* motivated to do it. Try finding an exer-cise buddy to keep you going, consider a personal trainer to kick-start your program, or get your partner to come with you for regular walks where you can talk about the day as you exercise.

- If your partner has weight to lose, encourage him to do so, too. Being overweight can affect male fertility and reduce the quality and quantity of his sperm count.[29]

- If you find that you need more advanced weight-loss help, or you feel that emotional eating is your underlying issue, turn to the next chapter on tackling stubborn problems for more ideas.

PCOS Weight-Gain Guidelines

If weight gain, not weight loss, is what you need, don't be tempted to reach for cookies and unhealthy junk food in order to increase your calorie intake. Try to resist these foods, as they fill you up and will prevent you from eating the more nutritious, fertility-boosting foods that your body and your future baby-to-be need. Aim to eat little amounts often, and consume plenty of healthy, fresh foods—especially fruits and vegetables and food rich in oils, such as fish, nuts, seeds, and olives.

Step Two: Get As Fit and As Well As You Can

Becoming as fit and as healthy as you possibly can involves both you and your partner exercising regularly, as well as getting the all clear from your doctor and getting checked for and treating any infections.

The Benefits of Exercise

For women with PCOS, exercise is particularly beneficial. Not only can it kick-start weight loss, but it has also been proven to help insulin and glucose control, which in turn means that your ovaries are encouraged to produce less testosterone, thus promoting hormonal balance and easing symptoms. Equally important, when symptoms of PCOS result in a loss of self-esteem, exercise can help you feel good about yourself—and when you feel good, you're less likely to eat unhealthy foods and more likely to feel positive about your fertility-boosting plan.

Exercise can also boost fertility. You don't have to be fit to be fertile, but it sure can help. If you're reasonably fit, this can improve your chances of conceiving. Habitual exercise can regulate your hormones and menstrual cycle in a beneficial way by helping you reach a healthy body weight and keeping stress levels down, therefore encouraging consistent ovulation.[30]

But don't overdo it: Training for more than 15 hours a week will have the opposite effect and inhibit ovulation.[31] Women who exercise to the extreme, such as gymnasts, dancers, and other athletes, can lose their menstrual cycle because of the reduction in body weight.

Exercise has lots of other benefits for you and your partner. For example, it does the following:

- Reduces stress

- Lowers blood sugar levels

- Promotes insulin efficiency

- Inspires good sleep patterns

- Boosts circulation

- Reduces the risk of heart disease and diabetes

- Improves blood supply to your reproductive organs

- Boosts your feeling of both mental and physical well-being

With all these benefits, it's no wonder that fitter people tend to feel more confident and sexy.[32, c]

Fitting Exercise into Your Life

A good, balanced exercise program provides three important benefits: stamina, strength, and flexibility. A woman needs all three to lift and carry a baby, run after a small child, and cope with the day-to-day stresses of motherhood. Plus, getting in shape at least three months before you conceive may make it easier to maintain an active lifestyle during pregnancy and actually enjoy those nine months, not to mention helping you get through labor. Strengthening your back muscles now, for example, can stave off lower-back pain later. And aerobic exercise can improve your mood and energy levels, not to mention help you achieve a healthy prepregnancy weight. You'll also be less vulnerable to the hormonal shifts that can make pregnant women irritable and send family and friends running for cover.

Great exercises to help get into shape for pregnancy include running, power walking, jogging, swimming, bicycling, and aerobics. Some of these are fairly strenuous, however, and shouldn't be taken up for the first time while pregnant, so be sure to begin well before you start trying to conceive. Then you can continue your routine when you're pregnant. For flexibility and stress relief, exercises such as tai chi, yoga, and Pilates are also good.

How Fit Are You?

Test yourself:

- Can you walk briskly for ten minutes without feeling exhausted?

- Can you walk up a flight of stairs without losing your breath?

Sit quietly and check your resting heart rate. Find your pulse where your wrist joins your hand, just below the thumb and about a half inch from the edge of your wrist. Count the beats for 20 seconds then multiply by three. If the results are under 70, you're pretty fit; 80–100 is okay;

over 100 isn't okay, and is a sign that you need to get in shape.

Aim for around 30 minutes of continuous exercise that works your large muscles and elevates your breathing and heart rate every day, or every other day. If you're a beginner, start with 10 minutes and gradually build to 30 minutes over a period of three to four months. Fitting exercise into your life is much easier if you find something you enjoy. Check out what your fitness options are. Could you walk to work instead of drive? How about taking up running or joining a fitness class? Do you enjoy swimming or cycling? Or would you enjoy something else, such as hip-hop dancing, yoga, or martial arts?

If you really hate to exercise and despise the gym, sports, or classes, why not take up walking? This activity is ideal because it doesn't really seem like exercise, but even 10 or 15 minutes a day can make a real difference. In fact, walking is highly recommended for women with PCOS. Dr. Robert Franklin believes that "walking is particularly good for PCOS patients. Not only is it great exercise, but it is a great way to de-stress and give you some time to yourself."

(*Note:* For all of the above activities, start slowly and don't push yourself too hard. You should always consult your doctor before starting any new exercise program.)

Visit Your Doctor for a General Checkup

If you want to try to have a baby, it's important that you visit your doctor for a general checkup, which should include the following:

• A blood-pressure test

• A urine check for infection and also for blood-sugar levels

- A Pap smear

- A blood-type test

- A discussion of any long-term health conditions, such as diabetes, and their implications for pregnancy

- A discussion of any medication you're taking to see if it's safe to take during pregnancy, and whether it could affect your fertility

- An investigation for silent genitourinary (GU) infections that could affect your chances of getting pregnant. You may not even know that you have one, as in some cases there are no noticeable symptoms. Ideally, before you try to get pregnant, you and your partner should have a screen test at a GU clinic for infections such as chlamydia, trichomoniasis, mycoplasma, ureaplasma, HIV, cytomegalovirus (CMV), rubella, Group B hemolytic streptococci, Gardnerella (bacterial vaginosis), and toxoplasmois. Your partner should also be tested for toxoplasmosis and CMV, which although not GU infections can also play havoc with fertility. If the sperm is infected even mildly, it can make all the difference between being able to help make a baby and not.

Your General Health

The preconception period is the ideal time to really focus on your general health and well-being. Do you wake up in the morning feeling energetic, or do you crawl out of bed feeling exhausted before the day has even begun? Do you rarely get ill, or are you always coming down with colds and infections? Is it easy for you to get around, or do you suffer from fatigue and/or mysterious aches and pains that slow you down? If it's the latter, these could be signs that your health isn't at the optimal level. Eating healthfully and exercising regularly may be all that you need to get you back on track, but if you don't feel as fit and healthy as you possibly can, do discuss this with your doctor.

The Age Issue

Are you over 35? The medical term for the mature mom (any woman who has a baby when she's over the age of 30) is quite intimidating: *elderly primigravida*. Although more and more women are having babies later in life, it's important to bear in mind that the 20s are considered to be our reproductive prime, with the least amount of fertility and health complications for mother and child.

Whether you have PCOS or not, at about the age of 35 most women start to become less fertile and may not ovulate every month, even though they still menstruate regularly. (A slight shortening of the monthly menstrual cycle is also common with age.) If you have PCOS and are having problems ovulating, clearly being over 35 isn't going to boost your chances, but try not to let this panic you. You can still raise your fertility levels with diet, exercise, health checks, and, if necessary, fertility treatment.

Contraception

You may be wondering why we're discussing contraception in a book about fertility! While you're getting as fit and as well as you can before trying to conceive, you need to use a form of contraception you can trust, but which will also allow your fertility to return quickly when you stop using it. If you have PCOS, what are your options?

1. **The combined Pill** is one of the most reliable forms of contraception and the treatment most likely to be offered by your doctor for PCOS symptoms such as irregular periods, acne, and hair loss. But what are the pros and cons when it comes to the effect on your fertility?

Studies have shown that it could cause a number of nutrient deficiencies, including vitamins B1, B2, B6, and B12; vitamins C and E; zinc; and folic acid.[33] As you'll see in Step Four (on page 36), all of these are essential fertility-boosting nutrients. You can ensure that you make changes in your diet and lifestyle to counteract the problems the Pill can cause. Women with PCOS who are on the Pill need to especially eat healthfully and exercise regularly and to take a good multivitamin and mineral to avoid nutritional deficiencies.

According to the British Medical Association Concise Guide to Medicines and Drugs, the Pill can also affect blood sugar balance: "Estrogens may also trigger the onset of diabetes mellitus in susceptible women, or aggravate blood-sugar control in diabetic women."[34] This isn't good news for women with PCOS, since the condition is already associated with insulin resistance (a precursor state to diabetes).[35] High levels of insulin stimulate the ovaries to produce large amounts of male hormones called *androgens*. Excess androgens are thought to stop the ovaries from releasing an egg, causing irregular or absent periods and subfertility.

When the Pill first came on the market, there was much concern about its long-term threat to fertility, but so far, that concern remains unproven, and most women ovulate within six to eight weeks after they withdraw from it. Indeed, there are some studies that suggest that the Pill can actually boost fertility, with some research suggesting that by preventing ovulation, it preserves your better-quality eggs for future use.[36]

Other Pill studies, however, give us a fuller picture of its effect on fertility and the significance of this for women with PCOS.[37-9] Some studies suggest that among previously fertile women who stop taking the Pill in order to conceive, the majority delivered a child within 30 months. These statistics seem to bode well, but it was found in another study of "older" childless women (between the ages of 30 and 35), that they experienced a marked delay when trying to conceive after coming off the Pill. Fifty percent of these women took a year longer to get pregnant—sometimes taking as long as 72 months—than those of the same age who had not been using the Pill.

Few women—especially ones over 35 with PCOS—want to risk waiting six years once they start trying to have a baby. More to the point, the study only looked at 30- to 35-year-olds; there have been no similar studies on women older than this, and logic would indicate that the figures probably wouldn't get better, but worse. Now add PCOS into the mix—a condition that further reduces your chances of conceiving—and the picture becomes quite a gloomy one.

So should you take the Pill? The choice, of course, is yours, but the chance that you could be one of those women who experiences a long delay in conceiving once you stop taking it would seem to suggest that switching to a more natural form of contraception as part of your preconceptual care routine is a good idea. If you're concerned, you might want to discuss with your doctor other contraceptive methods; or other treatments for irregular periods, hair loss, facial or body hair, or acne.

2. **The progesterone-only Pill** works by thickening the cervical mucus so that sperm can't get to the egg. If you miss a single dose, fertility can return within two days—and there isn't any evidence of a delay in fertility once you stop using it. However, some women with PCOS say that the progesterone-only Pill makes symptoms worse, and a study at the University of Southern California Medical School found that the progestin-only Pill increased the risk of insulin resistance and diabetes.[40] (Progestin is a synthetic version of progesterone.)

3. **Contraceptive injections,** such as Depo-Provera; and **implants,** such as Norplant, offer protection for anything between 8 and 12 weeks for injections, and up to three years for implants. They work by stopping ovulation and making your womb lining thinner and less likely to accept a fertilized egg. Your fertility and periods may take several months or years to return, even if you only ever had one injection or implant, and for this reason, they aren't the most sensible choice for women with PCOS.

4. **The IUD (intrauterine device)** is 98 percent effective, depending on which type is used. It's a small plastic device that works by causing a mild inflammation of the womb so that its lining won't allow a fertilized egg to implant. An IUD will also inhibit the sperm's ability to move. Fertility usually returns promptly after an IUD removal, but it's important that you're aware that there's always a risk of it causing pelvic infection while it's in place. If such

an infection were to reach your fallopian tube and cause scarring, the blockage could affect future fertility.

5. **Barrier methods** of contraception include the diaphragm, cervical cap, condom, and female condom. They work by stopping sperm from reaching the small passageway that runs through the center of the cervix. If used with spermicides, which work by killing sperm, they are approximately 97 percent effective.

Barrier methods are probably the best choice of contraception for women with a hormonal problem like PCOS, as they don't involve hormonal manipulation. In addition, your fertility will return as soon as you stop using them, which makes them the ideal choice of contraception for a couple following a preconceptual care program.

6. By learning to recognize your fertile time of the month, you can work out when to have intercourse to maximize or minimize your chances of pregnancy. This is the theory behind **natural family planning (NFP).**

With NFP, you time intercourse to coincide with ovulation if you want to get pregnant, and avoid it when you're ovulating if you don't. There are only a few days in each cycle when an egg is ripe for fertilization. A cycle is the time between the start of one period and the start of the next. To count the days of a cycle, start with the first day of the menstrual bleeding: This is day one. Continue counting until the first day of the next period, when you return to day one. An average cycle lasts around 28 days, although anything between 21 and 35 days is considered normal.

In a regular 28-day cycle, ovulation will normally take place around days 12 to 14 before the next period. There are various schools of thought, but it is generally held that if a couple is trying to get pregnant, they should make love at least every other day around ovulation. Sperm are capable of fertilizing an egg up to 48 hours after ejaculation, some even longer, and an egg can be fertilized for up to 24 hours after ovulation. This gives a window of around three to six days in the cycle, during which intercourse should take place if you want to get pregnant, or be avoided if you don't.

If you do have regular menstrual cycles, keep a record over a period of months so that you can assess those days when ovulation is most likely to occur, by subtracting 14 from your expected start date. There is some variation, but most doctors suggest that if you have a 28-day cycle, your fertile week would run from day 10 to 17.

This all sounds so simple, but in reality, it isn't. It's fine if your periods are regular, but what if you can't really predict your fertile week because your cycles change all the time? Most women don't have completely regular cycles, and the majority of women with PCOS have irregular or absent cycles, so even if periods do occur regularly, this isn't necessarily a definite indication of ovulation. If your periods are absent, NFP obviously isn't for you (see Chapter 3 for advice on how to restart your periods). Do bear in mind, though, that just because you aren't menstruating doesn't mean you can't get pregnant. Remember, ovulation occurs before your period starts.

When Are You Ovulating?

If you aren't sure whether or not you're ovulating, there are a number of ways in which you can determine whether and when you are.

Ovulation-predictor kits are available from your pharmacist and offer a simple method of predicting ovulation just before it happens by detecting a subtle change in hormone levels. However, generally for women with PCOS and irregular periods, they aren't reliable. (See Chapter 3 for more information and an explanation of the above.)

Check your cervical mucus: It can be thick, white or pale yellow, and sticky. As ovulation approaches, the mucus becomes more copious, clear, and elastic—a bit like an egg white.

Some women can tell when they're ovulating without any form of testing because they experience discomfort near the middle of their cycle for a day or so just before the egg is released, along with symptoms such as breast tenderness, increased libido, and a dull pain or ache in the ovary that's about to release an egg.

NFP is often recommended by preconceptual-care advisers as a form of contraception, but it isn't foolproof. New research has even suggested that there may not be any time in the month when it's safe to have sex. "It may be the case that for a large proportion of the female population, natural birth control is simply not an option," says Dr. Roger Pierson of the University of Saskatchewan, Canada, who led a study and whose findings were published in the medical journal *Fertility and Sterility* in July 2003. It also takes about four or five months to learn the method properly and become confident and comfortable with it, so if you really don't want to get pregnant right now, it's not a good choice.

Step Three: De-stress

"I'm a night nurse in a hospice, and it's sometimes really hard to switch off from the pain, loneliness, and suffering I see every day. Whenever I feel really tired and anxious, my symptoms get worse— especially the hair loss.

"I haven't had a regular period in years, I'm 30 next month, and I've been trying for a baby for two years. I went to my doctor to discuss my fertility, and he told me that I might have to consider changing jobs, as the nature of the work I do and the fact that I work nights is stressful both emotionally and physically. You see, stress may be making my symptoms worse and also be making it harder for me to get pregnant." — Jenny, 29 years old

If you have got PCOS, stress management is important. Recent research from the University of Birmingham and information published in the online journal *Genetics* has suggested that the high testosterone levels associated with PCOS could be caused by a fault in the way the body processes the stress hormone *cortisol*.

Cortisol, the active form of the hormone, can be turned into cortisone, the inactive form, by enzymes in the body. Researchers have found that some women don't have these enzymes, which means that their bodies can't process cortisol properly—thus, higher levels of testosterone are produced.

So watching your stress levels is of great significance if you have PCOS. And if you want to get pregnant, it's important, too. Why? Because too much stress not only triggers PCOS symptoms, it can also make them worse, including side effects such as weight gain and irregular periods, which, as we've seen, can both interfere with conception.

Dr. Rosalind Bramwell of the University of Liverpool and Dr. Robert Delman from the Roehamptom Institute, U.K., believe that stress is both an emotional and a physical state that has very real effects on a human's hormonal system—in particular, the output of sex hormones—due to its disturbance of the pituitary gland, which controls the process. It can also affect testosterone levels, interfering with ovulation, and, of course, making symptoms of PCOS worse.

Stress and Your Periods

Prolonged disturbance to your menstrual cycle may not always be due to PCOS, but could be due to the pressure you're under. It's not unusual to hear of women who've had problems trying to get pregnant for years, and who conceive once the pressure is lifted.

Studies show that extreme stress can stop ovulation.[41] For example, women going through bereavement or other kinds of trauma often stop having periods altogether. The women's hospital of the Berlin Charlottenburg in Germany found that out of approximately 2,000 couples being investigated for fertility in the late 1980s, in a quarter of all cases the cause was stress.

And it's not just extreme stress either—everyday events and experiences can all take their toll. For example, the prospect of a driving test can be enough to make you miss a period.

Stress and Fertility

Stress also hampers fertility because it produces unhealthy sperm and eggs, or both, and pregnancies created by damaged sperm or eggs usually result in early miscarriage.[42]

What's more, higher-than-normal levels of stress hormones can also affect your libido because they can have a domino effect on the hormones—estrogen and testosterone—that power your sex drive. Not having enough sex or, as some experts believe, not enjoying sex if you do, is a prime cause of infertility.

Stress can affect male fertility, too. It can influence a man's libido as well as his sperm. Research has shown that men under stress at work or home are more likely to have poor sperm quality and may experience poor fertility.[43]

Progressive fertility units such as the Beth Israel Hospital in Boston and the Harvard Behavioral Medicine Program have been including stress reduction in their programs for 15 years. "Our experience at the Division Behavioral Medicine in the Beth Israel Deaconess Medical Center (and this is backed up by research) is that women with long-term infertility may well increase their chances of conception when they reduce their levels of stress and depression," says Alice Domar, director of the Mind/Body Institute at the center.[44]

The International Europe survey of 2000 has identified stressful work as a major factor in infertility.[45] It seems that high public-contact jobs, and high-stress jobs such as flight attendant, teacher, or nurse, increase the risk of miscarriage.

Whatever the reason for your stress—be it anxiety about PCOS and/or your fertility, exhaustion from too much exercise, worries about your job, or being upset because of troubles in your relationship—you may very well find that this interferes with your health and fertility.

Stress is a fact of life, so you can't avoid it, but you can find ways to manage it. In fact, simply recognizing that you're stressed or anxious can be an important step.

Stress-Management Tips

1. Any stress management regime needs to begin with a **healthy eating plan** (see Step Four on page 36). Taking time to eat a balanced diet at regular mealtimes will ensure that your body remains healthy and able to cope during stressful times.

2. **Take a multivitamin and mineral.** It's your adrenal glands that produce the stress hormones—cortisol and adrenaline—and when you're under too much pressure, they start to wear down and overproduce not just cortisol and adrenaline, but testosterone, too. Excess cortisol, adrenaline, and testosterone will not only make PCOS worse, but will also drive your body toward irregular periods and subfertility. The adrenals rely on vitamins C, B5, B6, zinc, and magnesium, and these are rapidly depleted when you're under stress, so a good multivitamin and mineral every day makes sense.

3. **Get enough sleep**—even though women with PCOS are prone to suffer from a lack of it. Not getting enough quality sleep makes it harder to handle stress and affects quality of life, according to a poll by the U.S. National Sleep Foundation. In addition to raising stress hormones, research shows that sleep deprivation results in hormonal imbalance, therefore increasing the risk of infertility.[46] A good night's sleep is the best tonic you can have, but it's important to realize that quality, not quantity, is the key. A recent study at Brigham and Women's Hospital in Boston showed that a good night's sleep makes you feel happier and more relaxed, but those who had under six hours or over ten hours became irritable. Seven to eight hours seems ample for most people, but six hours of good-quality sleep beats a restless nine hours.

To encourage a good night's sleep, avoid eating, drinking, and exercising for at least two hours before you go to sleep. Try to stick to a regular bedtime, preferably before midnight, and a regular waking time. Keep fresh air circulating in your bedroom; the brain's sleep center works better with oxygen. Make sure your bedroom isn't too noisy, light, untidy, hot, or cold. A warm bath, perhaps with a few drops of lavender or neroli oil, can have a sedative quality. Simple relaxation techniques before you go to sleep, such as gentle stretching or meditation, can also help.

4. **Meditation** is a great way to lower both physical and mental stress. To try meditation by yourself, find a quiet place where you won't be interrupted. Make sure you're comfortable, and then start to imagine each part of your body from your toes to your scalp relaxing, while mentally repeating a neutral thought (try a color). When other thoughts break through the calm, just let them come and go. After ten minutes, open your eyes and sit quietly for a few moments before getting up.

Transcendental Meditation

Why not try transcendental meditation, which is thought to be up to eight times more beneficial to your health than other relaxation techniques. Training consists of a one-hour session where you're given a mantra to repeat over and over as you sit quietly. Follow-up classes fine-tune your technique. You should then meditate for 20 minutes twice a day, and the proven benefits include increased mental and physical alertness and better coping skills when under stress.

5. **Massage** can help. The sense of well-being you get from a rubdown can lower the amount of stress hormones, such as cortisol, circulating throughout your body. Either book a session with a qualified practitioner, or if you have time and think it would be fun, use a good book or a video to learn some simple techniques.

6. **Take up yoga.** "Mind," the U.K.'s leading mental-health charity, recommends yoga as the single most effective stress buster. Yoga has been around for thousands of years, and although its many famous fans have helped it become trendy now, its benefits

remain constant. The poses aim to bring your mind, body, and breathing together to improve posture and physical health and help you achieve a sense of calm.

7. **Think about how you react to stress** and identify those people and situations that trigger it. You can't avoid every trigger, but you don't have to invite them into your life.

8. **Use simple relaxation techniques to deal with short-term stress.** For example, if you get tense when stuck in traffic, try simple exercises such as tensing your muscles hard and relaxing them, or deep breathing for a count of ten, or daydreaming about a vacation. Other techniques include drinking calming herbal teas such as chamomile, having a good laugh, chatting with a friend, reading an interesting book, or listening to soothing music. Set aside 10 or 20 minutes a day to relax, no matter what.

9. The **exercise** you're doing in this preconceptual care stage is also great for beating stress. Not only does it stimulate the body's pituitary gland to release tension and give you a natural high, it also tires you out so that you sleep better no matter how much your mind is racing. Research also shows that regular exercise makes you less tense and better able to cope with stress.

10. **Try not to be a perfectionist.** Let the dishes sit in the sink a little longer, return that call tomorrow, and wear clothes you feel comfortable in. Learn to manage your time more effectively so that each day won't seem like such a struggle. Plan your day and prioritize what needs to be done. Tackle tasks one by one, and allow extra time for the unexpected.

11. **Breathe deeply.** You see, stress forces you to take shallow breaths that don't let your body get rid of tension the way a deep breath can. A large inhalation centers and calms the body, but most of us take tiny breaths. Practice this technique the next time you feel stressed: to a count of four, breathe in through your nose,

right down into your stomach, hold for one, then push the breath out again for a count of four.

12. **Simply talking to friends, family members, and partners can ease stress.** If you don't feel as if you have anyone you can talk to, a trained counselor can help you get in touch with your feelings and give you tips on stress management. You may also find that you get a great deal of support and encouragement from other women with PCOS. If you haven't already, think about joining a PCOS support group (you'll find contact details in the Resource Guide). Finally, don't forget that your very best friend and support is you. Instead of being your own worst enemy, be as nice to yourself as you are to your friends.

Step Four: Eat Fresh, Healthy Food Packed with Fertility-Boosting Nutrients

"My mom started seeing a nutritionist when her weight spiraled out of control, and to give her support I went to the meetings with her. To encourage her, I also cut down on saturated fat and sugar, increased my fruit and vegetable intake, and—most important of all—started eating breakfast and snacking regularly on healthy foods during the day so that I wouldn't have a massive chocolate binge on the way home from work. I also started taking a multivitamin and mineral. As if by magic, my periods— after being irregular for years because of PCOS—now appear every 28 or so days. In the next year or so, I want to start thinking of babies, and it's good to know that with regular periods and a healthy diet, I stand a very good chance of getting pregnant."
— Francesca, 29 years old

The foods you eat can improve your fertility, according to Dr. Margaret Rayman, Director of the MSc Course in Nutrition Medicine at the University of Surrey. What you eat affects every single cell and system in your entire body and is needed to produce healthy eggs (and sperm) for the development of your baby when you get pregnant. A healthy, balanced diet in the preconception period will not only boost your chances of having a healthy baby, but it will also help keep your weight down and your blood-sugar levels in balance. If your blood sugars aren't balanced, then your hormones, which control your fertility, won't work properly either.

Balancing Blood-Sugar Levels

The link between blood-sugar levels and hormone balance was first recognized by Dr. Katharina Dalton when she found that her patients who suffered from PMS saw that their symptoms were relieved by eating regularly. The "little and often" approach to eating prevents blood-sugar levels from dropping and stops adrenaline from being released. Adrenaline blocks the utilization of progesterone in the second half of the menstrual cycle, and this was causing symptoms of PMS.

The answer was to stabilize blood-sugar levels by getting patients to eat properly so that adrenaline didn't interfere with their hormone balance. Dalton's work has huge implications for fertility. If progesterone is blocked, it reduces the chances of conception, since this hormone is needed to maintain the womb lining at the start of a pregnancy.

There's also a clear link between blood-sugar balance problems and conditions such as PCOS, diabetes, poor eating habits, and excess weight. If your blood-sugar levels zoom up and down chaotically, not only will this affect your hormones, but it can also spark sugar cravings, food obsessions, and poor eating habits, which in turn can lead to weight gain.

Healthy eating can restore your blood-sugar and hormone balance, improve your energy levels, and help you lose weight, as well as addressing irregular periods and subfertility. "Eating a healthy, well-balanced diet of fresh, whole foods in combination with moderate exercise is," in the words of Helen Mason, senior lecturer in reproductive endocrinology at St. George's Hospital Medical School, London, "the first line of treatment for PCOS infertility patients."

Leading international nutritionist Dr. Gillian McKeith also believes that the food you eat is crucial. "In every clinical case I have come across with a female wishing to become pregnant and trying unsuccessfully, she has exhibited one major nutrient deficiency," she says. So by taking the time to eat a healthy diet, not only are you helping your PCOS, you're also boosting your fertility.

Your Healthy PCOS Diet

But what is a healthy diet for PCOS? It follows basic rules—the right amount of complex carbohydrates, moderate amounts of protein, sufficient essential fats, a minimum of saturated fats, and lots of water.

1. **Water** is an essential but often forgotten ingredient in a healthy eating plan. Water intake is vital for hormonal function, and you need to drink lots of it to keep your hormonal systems at their best. Try to drink at least one and a half quarts or six to eight glasses of fresh water a day.

2. To optimize your fertility, you should eat plenty of **unrefined complex carbohydrates**, which don't lead to a sudden rise in your blood-sugar levels. This means choosing whole-grain bread and pasta, instead of the refined white versions, which have been stripped of their valuable fiber content, and at least five servings of vegetables each day. Simple carbohydrates in the form of sweets, cakes, and white sugar can all produce a sudden rise in blood sugar, so it's important to avoid them.

Fruits are the exception here as they're a simple sugar, and they're packed with fertility-boosting nutrients. You shouldn't cut fruit out, but make sure you eat it with proteins, such as a few nuts or seeds or some low-fat yogurt, which can slow down the effect on blood sugar.

We need fiber to keep our digestive systems healthy, but it's also vital for our fertility because it can help keep our reproductive systems in optimal condition by helping clear out toxins and old hormone residues. It isn't difficult to increase your fiber intake, and you don't need to add bran to everything. Just eat more complex carbohydrates: whole-grain rice, bread, and pasta; and plenty of fruits, vegetables, beans, nuts, and seeds.

3. **Protein** is important for your fertility because it helps maintain blood-sugar balance and gives your body the even supply of amino acids it needs to build and repair cells and manufacture hormones. Since your body can't store protein the way it does carbohydrates and fat, you need a constant supply and should aim to eat some high-quality protein with every meal. Good sources of protein include low-fat dairy products, lean meat, eggs, legumes, beans, nuts, and seeds.

4. Unfortunately, **fat** in general has gotten a bad name, although it's the saturated fats found in meat and full-fat dairy products that are harmful. Essential fatty acids (EFA) found in nuts, seeds, and oily fish play a crucial role in fertility and the development of a healthy baby.[47–8]

Scientists have looked at their role in pregnancy and found that they're crucial for the brain, eyes, and nervous-system development of a growing baby. If you don't eat enough EFA, hormone production will also be compromised. It takes three months to build up your body's stores, so make sure you eat some every day. Good sources include evening primrose oil, flaxseed oil, and oily fish. Have a handful of nuts every day, or use a salad dressing made with a good quality nut or seed oil. The recommended daily dose is 1,000 mg flaxseed oil.

5. Finally, in addition to an adequate intake of every nutrient, a healthy, balanced diet should ensure that you consume specific **pro-fertility vitamins and minerals:**

— Infertile couples given *vitamin E* (200 IU per day for women and 100 IU per day for men), showed a significant increase in fertility in a preliminary trial.[49] Vitamin E's beneficial role in female reproductive health has since been backed up by more recent research.[50] Food sources include wheat germ, avocados, eggs, butter, whole-grain cereals, seeds, nuts, oily fish, and broccoli. The recommended daily dose is 300–400 IU.

— *Iron* deficiency should always be checked during infertility investigation, as taking iron is known to have helped women regain their fertility.[51] Even a subtle deficiency could contribute to infertility in women.[52] Iron supplements given together with vitamin C (which increases the absorption of iron) have resulted in a number of women with fertility problems becoming pregnant, including one woman who had undergone nine years of unsuccessful fertility treatment.[53-4] Your requirement for iron increases once you get pregnant. It's always better to get iron from food sources than from a supplement because of the risk of constipation and heartburn. Food sources include eggs, fish, powdered milk, dark green vegetables, lean red meat, and legumes.

— *Zinc* deficiency in women can lead to reduced fertility and an increased risk of miscarriage.[55] This mineral is vital for the development of unborn babies. Food sources include seafood, milk, whole grains, and dried fruit. Oysters are an especially good source of zinc. The recommended daily dose is 30 mg.

— Research has shown that women with low *manganese* levels are more likely to give birth to a baby with physical disabilities.[56] Food sources include tea, nuts, whole grains, and legumes. The recommended daily dose is 5 mg.

— Some previously infertile women have become pregnant after supplementing their diets with 100 mg of *PABA (para-aminobenzoic acid),* four times per day.[57] PABA is believed to increase the ability of estrogen to facilitate fertility.

— Another important vitamin for your fertility is *vitamin B12* (found in sardines, eggs, spirulina, and seaweed) according to a recent study.[58] Research has also shown that giving *vitamin B6* (good sources are avocados, lentils, and watermelon) to women who have trouble conceiving increases their fertility. In one study, 12 out of 14 women who had been trying to conceive succeeded after taking vitamin B6 daily for six months.[59] The recommended daily dose of each is 50 mg.

— Until recently, *folic acid* was just another B vitamin, but now conclusive research has shown its vital role in preventing spina bifida. Food sources include green beans, spinach, brussel sprouts, milk, and fruit. This is such an important nutrient that all doctors recommend taking it as a supplement in the preconception period. The recommended daily dose is 400 mcg.

— *Vitamin C* may also play a role. Research in the '70s showed that when given to women undergoing fertility treatment, it can help trigger ovulation, and recent research is confirming the nutrient's crucial role.[60] Vitamin C is found in raw fruits and vegetables, especially citrus fruits, black currants, kiwifruit, mangoes, red peppers, strawberries, and green sprouting vegetables such as brussels sprouts, watercress, and parsley. The recommended daily dose is 40 mg.

Vitamin C, along with vitamin E, may also play a role in preserving your fertility for longer. An interesting study was conducted at the department of pediatrics, obstetrics, and gynecology, faculty of medicine, University of Valencia, Spain.[61] It aimed to ascertain whether dietary supplementation with a mixture of vitamins C and E could prevent the maternal-age-associated decrease in egg quality in mice. The study showed promising results, with the age-related reduction in ovulation rate partially prevented by high doses of these vitamins.

Studies have yet to be done on humans, but these findings may have direct implications for preventing or delaying maternal-age-associated infertility.

— Supplementation with the amino acid *L-arginine* has been shown to improve fertilization rates in women with a previous history of failed attempts at in vitro (test tube) fertilization.[62]

— It's also important to have good levels of *vitamin A* at the point of conception because it's essential to the developing embryo, and in studies with animals, a deficiency of vitamin A produced newborns with birth defects. High doses of vitamin A aren't advised because this can also cause birth defects, but it seems that vegetable sources of beta-carotene, which your body can turn into vitamin A, are safe.[63–4, i]

Vitamin A (beta-carotene) is found in carrots, tomatoes, mangoes, pumpkins, cabbage, spinach, and broccoli. The recommended daily dose is up to 500 IU.

— In women, *selenium* deficiency is linked to miscarriage. Food sources include herring, tuna, whole wheat, broccoli, and garlic. The recommended daily dose is 100 mcg.

— According to research in the late '70s and again in the '90s, *magnesium* is one of the most important minerals affecting a woman's ability to conceive and the maintenance of the pregnancy itself.[65] Food sources include dairy products, nuts, vegetables, meat, cooked brown rice, and sunflower seeds. The recommended daily dose is 300 mg.

For Him

Your partner needs to ensure that he eats a wide range of nutrients, too. Research has shown that the following nutrients are of special importance to men because of their impact on sperm quality and quantity: vitamin A, B complex, magnesium, zinc, calcium, selenium, vitamin E, folic acid, and manganese.

Many nutrients important for fertility are quite fragile and easily destroyed by heating, cooking, and storage, so as a rule of thumb, try to eat your food as fresh and as close to its natural state—preferably organic—as possible. Avoid food that is processed and packed with chemicals, additives, and preservatives. Taking a good-quality daily multivitamin and mineral is also a good idea.

Women who take a daily multivitamin can double their chances of getting pregnant, say researchers from the University of Leeds. Researchers believe that taking a daily multivitamin can help produce better quality eggs.[66]

A study presented to the European Society of Human Reproduction and Embryology in July 2001 showed that in 215 women in Leeds undergoing in vitro fertilization (IVF) and taking a vitamin pill, the fluid surrounding the eggs was enriched with vitamins C and E, which the researchers believe can give the egg a crucial boost.

Gynecology senior registrar Dr. Sara Matthews, who lead the research, said: "My theory is that it might apply to anyone trying for pregnancy."

Supplements can be effective in rebalancing your hormones and improving health and fertility, but since all nutrients depend on each other to function properly, it's important to take a good multivitamin and mineral as the basic foundation, and then add in other individual nutrients on top to meet the required daily dose.

It's also important to remember that supplements are no substitute for a healthy diet. Dr. Ann Walker, a medical herbalist and nutrition research scientist based at the University of Reading's Hugh Sinclair Unit of Human Nutrition says, "There is no point in any medication or supplement coming in to correct symptoms that are caused by a bad diet and unhealthy lifestyle. It is important to get the diet and lifestyle healthy first, and then treat any outstanding health issues."

Before you go to the health-food store to buy supplements, it might be a good idea to see a dietitian or nutritionist, preferably one with an interest in fertility and, in an ideal world, experienced with PCOS patients. It pays to get a health professional to give you advice about diet and lifestyle. This adviser can check, using blood, sweat, or muscle testing, what nutrients you might lack, rather than having you buy a general prepregnancy or health-boosting formula that might not actually help you that much.

Your Fertility Eating Plan

The fertility buffet below was created by Vicky Chudleigh, state registered dietitian from Addenbrookes Hospital in Cambridge, U.K., to show that eating well doesn't have to be boring—and we've used that attitude to create the seven-day menu plan that follows for you.

The Fertility Buffet

APPETIZERS

Crêpes topped with smoked salmon and horseradish
Crostinis topped with pesto and roasted red peppers
Sunflower, pumpkin, sesame-seed, and brazil-nut bread
Extra-virgin olive oil with Parmesan for dipping

PLATTERS

A selection of cold and cured meats
A selection of fish sticks, mini crab cakes
    and sweet chili dip, and calamari
Goat cheese, thyme, and tomato tart

SALADS

Cucumber, fennel, celery, and chicory salad
A pasta salad with shredded watercress, baby spinach,
    and pesto
Sliced beefsteak tomatoes with basil dressing

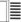
FRUIT KEBABS

Dacquoise (a delicate combination of almond
    meringue with cream and an apricot sauce)
Chocolate mousse
A selection of European cheeses and crackers
Chocolate-covered brazil nuts

The sunflower, pumpkin, and sesame-seed bread contains
vitamin E, which is claimed to be an aphrodisiac because of
its effects on boosting circulation. It's also an antioxidant and
needed for fertility. Brazil nuts and mini crab cakes are both
excellent sources of selenium, which is required for sperm
motility. Selenium also minimizes the risk of miscarriages.

All the other items on the menu were selected for their
fertility-boosting qualities. For example, spinach, together
with dark green leafy vegetables, provides the folate (another
name for folic acid) required to reduce the risk of neural tube
defects in a developing baby. Cheese contains calcium,
zinc, and vitamin A, which are all needed for healthy reproduction and libido.

A Week of PCOS Fertility-Boosting Menus

You can drink unlimited herbal teas and pure water with these
menus.

DAY ONE

Breakfast: A poached egg on whole-grain toast, and a glass of fresh-
squeezed apple juice (if you have a juicer; if not, have orange juice)

Mid-morning: A pear and six almonds

Lunch: A grilled chicken breast; a small baked potato; and a large "rainbow" salad with red peppers, carrots, red onions, spinach, and lettuce, sprinkled with sunflower and flaxseeds

Mid-afternoon: A small bar of organic dark chocolate and a glass of organic skim milk or fruit juice diluted with water

Dinner: Kebabs made with tofu or salmon, onion, peppers, and broccoli; brown basmati rice; a green salad; and stewed dried apricots with a little yogurt

DAY TWO

Breakfast: Oatmeal made with skim or soy milk and sprinkled with chopped brazil nuts, dried apricots, and dried figs; and a glass of fresh-squeezed apple juice

Mid-morning: A large slice of melon and a handful of mixed seeds with raisins

Lunch: Cheese or shrimp-salad platter with whole-grain pita bread, and fruit cobbler with low-fat ice cream

Mid-afternoon: A glass of soy milk and crackers

Dinner: Mixed seafood or tofu paella, a green salad, and a fresh-fruit salad

DAY THREE

Breakfast: Muesli or granola with extra flaxseeds and wheat germ sprinkled on it, and a glass of fresh-squeezed pineapple juice

Mid-morning: A glass of skim organic or soy milk and an apple

Lunch: Three-bean chili, a small baked potato or whole-grain rice, and onion and mint salad

Mid-afternoon: A handful of dried apricots or figs with five brazil nuts

Dinner: Seafood, chicken, or vegetarian-sausage pizza on a whole-grain crust, piled high with freshly cut vegetables and tomato sauce; a green salad; and sliced mango with lime juice

DAY FOUR

Breakfast: A bowl of mixed berries with chopped nuts, flaxseeds, and low-fat yogurt topping; and a glass of fresh-squeezed apple juice

Mid-morning: An apple and sunflower seeds

Lunch: A mozzarella, avocado, and tomato salad with lemon juice and flaxseed-oil dressing; a whole-grain roll; and a fruit salad

Mid-afternoon: A glass of skim milk or diluted fruit juice and a whole-grain fruit scone

Dinner: Chicken or tofu stir-fry with garlic, ginger, soy sauce, and lots of crunchy vegetables (such as carrots, broccoli, onions, peppers, green beans, and baby corn); whole-grain rice; and a small bar of dark chocolate

DAY FIVE

Breakfast: Lean bacon or tofu sausages, scrambled eggs, and a glass of fresh-squeezed apple juice

Mid-morning: A low-fat pretzel snack mix

Lunch: A bowl of vegetable soup sprinkled with flax and pumpkin seeds and a tuna or hummus sandwich on whole-grain bread

Mid-afternoon: An apple, three dried apricots, and a handful of walnuts

Dinner: Spiced lentils, whole-grain rice or pitas, a green salad, and fresh pineapple

DAY SIX

Breakfast: A boiled egg, whole-grain toast, and fresh-squeezed apple juice

Mid-morning: A glass of skim or soy milk and five brazil nuts

Lunch: Grilled fish, a baked potato, and a mixed "rainbow" salad

Mid-afternoon: A small muffin and an apple

Dinner: Green or red Thai curry (choose fish, chicken, or tofu), brown basmati rice, and a mixed-fruit salad with chopped nuts, seeds, and yogurt topping

DAY SEVEN

Breakfast: Toasted whole-grain English muffin, lean bacon or tofu sausage, ketchup (optional), and fresh-squeezed apple juice

Mid-morning: A small bunch of grapes and a handful of mixed nuts

Lunch: Grilled fish, chicken breast, or meat-substitute fillet (such as Quorn); and roasted mixed vegetables (roast peppers, onions, sweet potato, carrots, zucchini, and asparagus, sprinkled with olive oil and lots of crushed garlic, until tender)

Mid-afternoon: A glass of organic skim or soy milk and one small cookie

Dinner: A mixed salad with greens, crisp vegetables (onions, peppers, carrots, peas), cheese cubes, cashew nuts, beets, sliced hard-boiled eggs; hot garlic bread; and dark-chocolate mousse with raspberries

Step Five: Detox Your Lifestyle

There are many things in our day-to-day lives that can make the symptoms of PCOS worse, and anything that makes irregular periods worse will, of course, make it harder for you to get pregnant. There are now more than 300 chemicals that didn't exist 50 years ago, which can collect in your body, rob you of nutrients, and interfere with your hormonal health.[67]

Every day, a sea of hormone-disturbing toxins surrounds us. They're in cigarette smoke; pesticides and herbicides in our soil; chemicals and additives in the food we eat; contaminants in the water we drink; solvents, plastics, and adhesives; as well as all the toxins we absorb through our skin from makeup, hair dyes, and household cleaning products. Our bodies don't need or want any of these chemicals and have to work hard to process (metabolize) them and get rid of (detoxify) them through the liver, kidneys, lymph, and digestive systems. In the process of metabolizing and detoxing, our bodies also lose vital nutrients—which we need to feel healthy, beat the symptoms of PCOS, and boost fertility.

These toxins have also been linked to birth defects and hormonal disruption so great that some of them are now called *GED* or *general endocrine disrupters*. They could be interfering with your ability to conceive due to the damage they cause to your ovulation cycle and possibly your eggs, as well as to your partner's sperm production. "The cause of many infertility cases (up to 20 percent) remains unexplained," says Dr. John Sussman, fellow of the American College of

Obstetricians and Gynecology and founder of the "Preparation for Pregnancy" program at the New Milford Hospital, Connecticut. "Some think low-level exposure to toxins may eventually be found to be the culprit."

But it's not all doom and gloom—you can detox your lifestyle in simple ways to promote hormonal balance and fertility.

Keep Your Liver, Kidneys, and Lymph System Happy!

These organs function as your body's own detoxing powerhouse, and by keeping them healthy, you can help your body flush out harmful toxins and process old hormones so that they stop causing imbalances (for more on liver protection, see page 90 in Chapter 3). Keep your kidneys happy by drinking lots of pure water, balancing your protein intake with low glycemic-index (GI) carbs (foods that cause a gradual, less pronounced rise in blood sugar), and keeping your lymph system in good order with regular self-massage and exercise.

Smoking

Fertility experts agree that cigarettes and alcohol can be damaging. The advice to you and your partner is to give up smoking— or at the very least, cut down.

More than 600 chemicals are allowed in cigarettes, revealed a U.K. report published in 2000 by then-Health Secretary Alan Milburn. Smoking is a significant anti-nutrient—it actually reduces the level of vitamin C in the bloodstream. Smokers also have high levels of cadmium, a toxic heavy metal that can stop the utilization of zinc needed for a healthy menstrual cycle.

Scientists at Massachusetts General Hospital in Boston have found that smoking can trigger infertility in both men and women.[68] Other studies confirm that women who don't smoke are twice as likely to get pregnant as women who do.[69] Cigarettes reduce estrogen levels, which cuts down on the number of fertile years a woman has left to conceive, causes irregular periods, and makes eggs and cervical mucus less hospitable to sperm. In short, the more you smoke, the less likely you are to conceive.[70] In fact, women whose mothers smoked during their pregnancy are less likely to conceive compared with those whose mothers didn't.[71] So strong is the evidence that although there isn't an official antismoking policy from the U.K.'s Human Fertilization and Embryology Authority (HFEA), they strongly advise against it when undergoing fertility treatment. And it isn't unheard of for individual fertility clinics or specialists to refuse fertility treatment if their clients are heavy smokers.

This behavior damages almost all aspects of sexual, reproductive, and children's health, according to a February 2004 report by the British Medical Association (BMA). It's one of the major causes of impotence in men, is responsible for up to 5,000 miscarriages a year, reduces the chances of successful IVF, and is implicated in cases of cervical cancer.

The BMA is calling for tough antismoking measures, including help for pregnant women to avoid secondhand smoke. The report concludes that the damage inflicted by smoking is evident throughout reproductive life—from puberty to middle age. Not only can it keep people from starting a family, the report says, it can also damage their children. The BMA also states that smoking reduces the chances of a woman conceiving by up to 40 percent per menstrual cycle, and those who continue the habit during pregnancy are three times more likely to have a low birth-weight baby. There's also evidence that it may increase the risk of certain birth defects, such as cleft lip and palate. Women who inhale cigarette smoke have also been found to produce smaller volumes of lower-quality breast milk; while secondhand smoke is linked to sudden infant death syndrome (SIDS), premature birth, respiratory infection in children, and the development of childhood asthma.

Dr. Vivienne Nathanson, the BMA's head of science and ethics, said: "The sheer scale of damage that smoking causes to reproductive and child health is shocking. Women are generally aware that they should not smoke while pregnant, but the message needs to be far stronger. Men and women who think they might want children one day should [throw away] cigarettes. And we're not just talking about having children. Men who want to continue to enjoy sex should forget about lighting up, given the strong evidence that smoking is a major cause of male sexual impotence."

Deborah Arnott, director of antismoking charity Action on Smoking and Health (ASH), said: "The BMA report clearly shows the devastating impact of smoking on generations to come. Stopping smoking should be the number one priority for anyone who wants to have children. This is important not just to increase the chances of conception but also to give your child the best start in life."

Alcohol

Alcohol can also interfere with hormonal health. Research has shown that women who drink heavily can stop ovulating and menstruating and take longer to conceive. A study in the British Medical Journal in 1998 states categorically that women should avoid alcohol when trying to conceive. Alcohol may prevent enough progesterone being produced by the egg capsule, and progesterone is one of the major players in ensuring that a pregnancy is carried to term. Even moderate drinking is linked to an increased risk of infertility in some women.[72] In one preliminary study, there was a reduction of greater than 50 percent in the probability of conception in a menstrual cycle during which participants consumed alcohol.

We would suggest that if you have PCOS and are trying to bring your symptoms under control and boost your fertility, that you only drink alcohol in moderation (say, one glass of wine, liquor, or beer a day). Any more than that could have a harmful effect on your fertility. There are many lower-alcohol wines and liquors available today, as well as an increasing number of organic options.

It's not just you who needs to cut down—your partner does, too. A man can wipe out his sperm count for up to three months after a single heavy drinking session, according to Anthony Harsh, andrologist at Whipps Cross Hospital, U.K. This is because alcohol reduces the level of vital sperm-making hormones, and preconceptual care experts often insist that a man who wants to father a healthy child should stop drinking for at least three months before trying to get his partner pregnant.

Caffeine

You might also want to think about cutting down on the amount of caffeine in your diet. Drinking one to one and a half cups of coffee per day in one study, and about three or four cups per day in other studies, has been associated with delayed conception in women trying to get pregnant.[73,74-5] In another study, women who drank more than one cup of coffee per day had a 50 percent reduction in fertility, compared with women who drank less.[76] In another, even drinking three cups of decaffeinated coffee per day was associated with an increased risk of spontaneous abortion, and other research suggests that caffeine consumption compounded the negative effects of alcohol consumption on female fertility.[77-9, d]

Caffeine is found in regular coffee, black tea, green tea, some soft drinks, chocolate, and many over-the-counter pharmaceuticals. While not every study finds that caffeine reduces female fertility—both the U.S. National Institutes of Health and the American Heart Association suggest that drinking two cups of tea a day can reduce the risk of heart disease—many doctors recommend that women trying to get pregnant avoid caffeine or cut down.[80] So, overall, it seems that although you don't need to eliminate coffee, tea, chocolate, and colas altogether, you do need to cut down to no more than one or two cups a day, or switch to herbal or fruit teas.

Medications

Medications that you or your partner may take can also interfere with your fertility, and it's important that you're aware of their effects. When in doubt, if you need to take any kind of prescription drugs, talk to your doctor about the impact on your fertility. It's thought that commonly prescribed painkillers, such as ibuprofen, ketoprofen, and naproxen, may increase the risk of miscarriage. "Until we know more, these drugs should be avoided," says Professor James Driffe from the Royal College of Obstetricians and Gynaecologists in London.

Doubts have also been cast over the safety of acetaminophen. Low-dose aspirin, however, seems to be an exception, according to a 2001 study at the Institute of Health Sciences in Oxford, and may actually have a beneficial effect. But this area hasn't been researched widely, and further studies are needed to confirm the findings. The Royal College of Obstetrics and Gynaecology still advises that women concerned about their fertility check with their doctor before taking aspirin, acetaminophen, or any kind of painkiller.

Detox Your Food

If you have PCOS and are concerned about your fertility, it really is important to make sure that what ends up on your plate is as fresh and nutritious as possible. You need all the nutrients you can get to beat your symptoms and boost your fertility . . . and that means avoiding food that's been chemically treated.

Chemicals, pesticides, and preservatives used on food to keep them pest-free or make them last longer, taste different, or look different can build up over time.[81] Xenoestrogens (or synthetic estrogens) are environmental toxins derived from pesticides and plastics—we eat them in our food, drink them in our water, and store them in our body fat; and they can have a negative effect on our hormones.

We highly recommend that you and your partner eat organic food whenever possible. Organic food often contains higher levels of nutrients and is free from chemical pesticides, herbicides, and artificial fertilizers. To cut the cost of going organic, you could either join a community supported agriculture group (CSA), where you purchase a share of a season's harvest from local farmers so that you get fresh fruits and vegetables from local producers throughout the growing season, or you could visit your local farmers' market. If going organic isn't practical for you, there are ways you can protect yourself against xenoestrogens:

- If you can't eat just organic fruits and vegetables, at least always wash all fruits and vegetables thoroughly.

- Drink at least six glasses of water a day—add fruit juice if this gets boring—and filter your water. Use a stainless-steel filtration system fitted under your sink, if possible, not a plastic one.

- Reduce your intake of fatty animal products (meat and dairy), since xenoestrogens accumulate in fat.

- Never heat food in plastic containers and don't wrap food in plastic—the plastic contains toxins that can be absorbed by your food.

- Think brown—go for unrefined complex carbohydrates (brown rice and whole-grain pasta and bread). Avoid white bread, pasta, biscuits, cakes, and refined foods.

- Eat a leafy, green vegetable a day. Cruciferous vegetables such as broccoli, cauliflower, and cabbage can boost the liver's ability to detoxify harmful chemicals.

Detoxing Your Life

At home and at work, we're all exposed to toxins and health risks that could pose a threat to our fertility. For example, research shows that women who are exposed to heavy metals and chemicals (such as the following) often have problems with their menstrual cycle, experiencing hormone imbalances and miscarriages and taking longer to get pregnant:[82]

1. **Lead** is a toxic heavy metal that's naturally present in the earth, but we get exposure to it from lead pipes. Lead has been used in the past to induce abortion, and women who live in lead-polluted areas have a higher level of miscarriage.[83] Toxic lead exposure is also associated with birth defects and delayed development.[84] It's damaging to men, too: According to a 1991 study, of all the toxic metals, lead seems to pose the greatest threat to male fertility.[85] Research shows it can reduce sperm count, increase malformed sperm, and make sperm sluggish.

2. **Cadmium** also negatively affects male and female fertility, according to research.[86] It's an inorganic poison present in tobacco smoke that accumulates in the body and blocks vital fertility-enhancing nutrients such as zinc.

3. **Aluminum** can also seriously compromise nutritional status and therefore impact your fertility.[87] The main sources of aluminum are antacids, deodorants, antiperspirants, anticaking ingredients found in powdered milk, aluminum cookware, soft-drink cans, and foil.

4. **Mercury** is a heavy, toxic metal that now contaminates the air, soil, and water in many parts of the world. Traces of mercury can be found in pesticides, dental fillings, and fish (especially tuna). The saying "mad as a hatter" came about because people who made top hats used to polish them with mercury, and many of the "hatters" were poisoned by it. Mercury is extremely toxic, and studies show it can affect fertility.[88] This may be because the metal accumulates in the pituitary gland, which is vital for stimulating the production of sex hormones, and also because, according to experiments on mice in 1983, it appears to build up in the ovaries themselves. Other research links mercury with painful and irregular periods, reduced fertility rates, and premature birth.

Mercury is implicated in miscarriage for workers who are exposed to it in their profession, such as dentists and factory workers who deal with mercury compounds. Women dentists have a higher rate of miscarriage, and female dental assistants who are exposed to mercury through the fillings they handle have been found to be less fertile than female dentists who don't come into contact with the metal.[89] Recent research urges for the connection between mercury exposure and infertility in both men and women to be further investigated.[90-1]

If the fillings in your teeth are dark gray or silver, they contain mercury and other metals mixed together into what's called a *dental amalgam*. Unfortunately, mercury is poisonous, and vapors leach out of our fillings and into our body all the time, especially when we drink something hot, such as tea or coffee; when we brush our teeth; and when we chew gum. A study of several hundred research papers and clinical reviews suggests that mercury stored in our body may cause a wide variety of symptoms, including allergies, fatigue, mood disorders, flulike symptoms, menstrual problems, reduced sperm count, ovulation disorders, and miscarriage.[92-5] The use of dental amalgams has been banned in both Sweden and Austria on health grounds. In Japan and Germany, although not prohibited by law, there is a high level of awareness, and amalgam fillings are rarely used. In the U.K., the British Dental Association hasn't officially accepted that they're a health hazard, but a handful of private dentists are willing to help patients replace them with a safer alternative.

Checklist for Avoiding Reproductive Toxins

All the chemicals and other toxic substances that we absorb in our daily life can collect in our system, make symptoms of PCOS worse, and damage our fertility. There is a clear link between reproductive toxins and infertility, so it makes sense to avoid possible sources of contamination. First, see if your work or home exposes you to toxic metals, and then look for other ways to detoxify your body:

1. **Eat nutritious food and supplement wisely.** Following a cleansing diet as outlined above, avoiding alcohol, and eliminating cadmium from smoking and exposure to secondhand smoke—all of which can have a toxic effect on the body—are the best ways to

avoid toxin damage.[96] You may also want to take specific nutrients (see Diet and Detox box on page 60) to help eliminate the toxins from your system.

2. Michel Odent, the famous French gynecologist who introduced birthing pools and homelike birthing rooms, believes that **losing excess body fat** will help, since that's where we store toxins. If you're trying to lose weight, this can be another great motivator.

3. **Avoid aluminum** kitchenware, foil, and foods and antacids containing aluminum additives.

4. **Avoid lead.** Check if your water supply has lead pipes, as the metal can leach into the water just by standing in the pipes overnight. If you have lead pipes, allow your faucet to run for a minute first thing in the morning. Use cold water, not hot, because lead dissolves more easily into hot water. Also, use a filter for all your water, including cooking, hot drinks, and so on.

Wherever possible, avoid lead-polluted air; for example, don't stand around outdoors in heavy traffic areas, and close car windows when going through tunnels.

4. **Check the labels of toiletries and cosmetics.** Be especially wary of the aluminum in deodorants and antiperspirants; instead, use natural products.

5. **Refuse mercury-containing dental fillings,** and, when possible, have existing ones replaced with nontoxic alternatives. (Also watch out for high levels of mercury in canned tuna.)

6. **Check what chemicals and toxins you may be exposed to at work.** Carbon disulfide, used in several manufacturing processes, such as the production of plastics, has been linked to sexual dysfunction in both women and men. Many pesticides and herbicides are known reproductive toxins, so people working in gardens, parks, plant nurseries, and farms are at risk. Fertility problems in men and

women have been linked to exposure to specific substances on the job, such as anesthetics (affecting health workers such as nurses and veterinarians), traffic fumes and cheap paint (laborers), solvents (dry cleaning and laboratory staff), and glycol ethers (workers in electronics manufacturing).

7. **Limit your time spent at visual display unit (VDU) screens.** One study showed that women who spend more than 20 hours a week in front of a VDU screen, such as a television or computer monitor, have twice as many miscarriages as non-VDU workers.[97] Research on the impact of VDUs on reproductive health is still ongoing and no conclusions have been drawn, but if you do work in front of a screen, the tips below can help to reduce the impact.[98]

Computer Protection Tips

- Take regular breaks from the screen, at least five minutes every half hour.

- Switch the VDU off, rather than using the screensaver, when you're not using it

- Sit as far away from the computer as you can, while still being able to sit comfortably and see properly.

- According to the Institute de Recherches en Geobiologie at Chardonne in Switzerland, which has investigated the effects of radiation of a variety of plants, a cactus called Cereus peruvianus will help absorb some of the VDU's electromagnetic radiation

- An ionizer on top of your desk may help

8. **Check what toxins you may be exposed to in your own home.** Try not to use pesticides in your garden, and have your house treated for woodworm and termites when you aren't staying there.

Treat your pets or your house for bugs with natural herbal sprays or garlic. Be careful if you're decorating your home, and avoid solvent-based paints and turpentine. Buy solvent-free paints instead, and minimize the amount of chemicals you use in your home, such as polishes, bleach, detergents, and air fresheners. Try to buy natural products, or use tried-and-true cleaners such as vinegar, baking soda, or borax.

9. **Devices that emit electromagnetic radiation**, such as VDUs, televisions, cell phones, radios, and microwaves, should also be used with caution, and kept as far away from your bedroom as possible.

Diet and Detox

According to research by Foresight, "The preferred method of detoxification must undoubtedly be nutritional since it does not have the same potential for adverse side effects as drugs, which can remove essential elements as well as toxins."[99]

Research backs this up. A judicious choice of food can counteract toxic substances.[100] For example, when humans consume fish that have absorbed mercury from contaminated water, selenium can act as a natural antidote for mercury poisoning.[101] Some vegetables can accumulate cadmium from contaminated soil, but the zinc found in a variety of nuts and the vitamin C in oranges and bell peppers can inhibit absorption.[102] In addition, calcium neutralizes both lead and aluminum toxicity.[103]

Antioxidants are protective substances that patrol the body, mopping up toxins.[104] Research has shown how powerful they can be in removing these substances from the body. The antioxidant vitamins A, E, and C (as well as selenium) all have powerful detoxing effects.[105] Vitamin A helps activate the enzymes needed for detoxification.[106] In one study, vitamin C, along with zinc, reduced blood lead levels in psychiatric out-patients.[107] This nutrient has also been shown to lower cadmium levels in birds. Vitamin E is such a good detoxifying agent that those with the highest intake of vitamin E (along with vitamin C) have the lowest rates of cancer and heart disease. It may also reduce lead poisoning.

As an antioxidant, selenium protects against a wide variety of degenerative diseases, including liver disease.[108] Another beneficial supplement is sodium alginate.[109] This naturally occurring sea product is effective in helping remove toxic metals. Sulfur can be important too,[110–11] and garlic, cruciferous vegetables (brussel sprouts, cabbage, cauliflower, and broccoli), and eggs are good sources of nutritional sulfur. In studies done with mice, cruciferous vegetables have inhibited the induction of toxic overload and cancer. Researchers speculate that the phytochemicals in them, called *isothiocyanates,* help the body produce enzymes that destroy toxins.[112]

Step Six: Ask Yourself If You're Ready

Emotional health is as important for fertility as your physical condition. We've seen how your body is unlikely to ovulate if you aren't eating properly, and as we saw in the earlier section on stress, in a similar way, your sex hormones can fail to function properly if you're unhappy or distressed.

Stresses that have been found to suppress ovulation and menstrual-cycle functioning include low self-esteem, poor body image, and negative or ambivalent feelings about a relationship or the prospect of motherhood. Research has even shown that, in some cases, women who don't ovulate can often be more tense and anxious and have lower self-esteem compared to ovulating women.[113–14]

With the latest scientific research showing how emotional and psychological factors can be barriers to conception, finding ways to reconnect with your inner self and really focusing on what having a child means to you can be a healing process. Niravi Payne, internationally recognized leader in mind-body fertility and founder of the Whole Person Fertility Program in Brooklyn, New York, uses exercises, meditations, visualizations, and journal writing to help her clients topple any emotional barriers that may be behind their difficulty in conceiving. Payne recognizes that there are certain conditions, such as PCOS, that can prevent a pregnancy, but says, "I have found that the vast majority of reproductive difficulties are responsive to mind-body fertility therapy."

Without a doubt, the state of your mind and your body are connected (why else do you always come down with a cold when you feel stressed?). This isn't in any way to blame you for having PCOS—we want to emphasize that you, your partner, and your body aren't in any way to blame if you have problems getting pregnant. But by becoming more aware of the connection between how you feel and what happens in your body, you may be able to influence your ability to conceive by making changes in your life.

"When my twin brother died in a car crash, I was 15, and it felt as if my arms and my legs had been cut off. I somehow stumbled through school and college and into the workplace, but a part of me was deeply wounded. I had a few disastrous relationships, but then I met a guy who made me feel happy for the first time in years. We got married and started trying for a baby. When nothing happened, my doctor explained that I had PCOS and would need fertility drugs. I had three cycles of Clomid, but nothing happened.

"Then my husband's parents died within a few months of each other, and we both felt that we needed to take a break from the treatment. My husband was very open with his grief, and I watched him feel the hurt and gradually take steps to move forward with his life—something I'd never done. For the first time, I sat down in a heap and cried about all the hurt, the pain, and the loss I felt when I was 15 and didn't have the emotional resources to cope with the enormity of it all. It sounds strange,

but it felt good to let go, as if I'd been waiting for this moment, and now I could breathe again.

"A few months later, I got pregnant without the help of Clomid or any other drug. You can say it was luck, but I really feel that until I'd let my pain and sadness for my brother go, my body wasn't ready to let a new life begin." — Jane, 32 years old

What do you feel about the prospect of motherhood? Do you think that you'll make a good mother? Have negative feelings about yourself contributed to fertility problems? Are you ready to raise a child? It does seem that your body has a built-in mechanism to stop you from getting pregnant at times when you don't feel secure or ready for a baby. After all, if there are areas of your life that you're struggling with, these can be so much harder to cope with when a baby arrives.

How Positive Are You?

It isn't always easy to know if you're under emotional strain, but when asked to describe a positive state of mind, psychologists include the following:

- Feeling okay and reasonably content: When you wake up in the morning, how do you feel? How many times do you laugh during the day? Do you ever feel happy for no reason? Can you think of the future without feeling anxious?

- Having stable moods and not being on a constant emotional roller coaster: How would you describe your general mood during the day? Is it fairly even, or will the least little thing get you really angry?

- Being able to connect with others, but also being happy in your own company: Do you have people in your life—perhaps a partner, a friend, or a relative— who you can open up to, or do you dread meeting people? Do you enjoy your own company, or do you hate being alone?

- Being able to give and receive love and affection: Is it easy and natural for you to express physical affection?

- Feeling your emotions fully and being able to manage them: Is it easy for you to allow yourself to feel strong emotions? Can you face difficult emotions such as anger, or do you fear them?

- Enjoying your relationships at home and work: Would you say that your relationships in general are positive, or are they strained? Do you enjoy your job? What's your home life like?

- Enjoying life's simple pleasures, such as food, sex, and exercise: Do you like your own body? Do you enjoy sex? Do you enjoy food and drink? Are you interested in many aspects of life and the world around you?

Everybody is different, and there's no right or wrong response to the questions above, but if you suspect that right now you aren't feeling as good about yourself or your life as you could, you may want to take stock. What do you need from the different areas of your life? Perhaps you could talk it over with someone you can trust, such as a friend, family member, or counselor.

Is the Clock Ticking?

"For seven years now, we've been trying for a baby. I'm in my early 30s, so I have time, but I can't help thinking that something is wrong with me. My partner and I are desperate for a baby, and I thought getting pregnant would be so easy. Well, it was for all my friends, but it wasn't for me. The thought that I might be infertile crosses my mind, but I keep pushing it away.

It makes me feel so depressed. I've recently been diagnosed with PCOS, and I'm not sure whether this makes me feel better or worse. I just want to know if I'll ever get to be a mother." — Sally, 32 years old

You can't slow down or stop the biological clock, but this doesn't mean that you have to be pressured by it. While it's true that you're working under a deadline, and 35 does seem like a crucial turning point for women with PCOS, it's vital that you don't panic. Panic won't help you make the best decision, and if you decide that you *do* want to conceive, it won't help you get pregnant either. If fears about your fertility and anxiety over whether or not you want or can have a baby are taking over your life, it's important that you visit your doctor or seek other advice and support. (See also the section on biological-clock anxiety on page 182.)

Step Seven: Enjoy Your Sex Life

"Sex really did lose magic and appeal when we started trying for a baby. At first we laughed about my calling John at work and saying, 'Come home now—I'm ready and waiting!' but as the months passed and nothing seemed to work, it actually got harder and harder to feel sexy. I just started thinking of sex as a mechanical process, rather than as a way of giving and receiving pleasure. I think John felt the same—it got more and more difficult for him to have erections. That, of course, made me feel that he didn't find me attractive. I didn't think that it might have something to do with the fact that in concentrating on having a baby, we'd neglected our relationship. Later, he told me that he felt like a sperm donor, not a husband." — Janet, 36 years old

If all you can think about is making a baby, sex can lose its spontaneity. No specific research has been done, but it does seem logical from conclusions drawn by other studies that enjoying lovemaking—and especially having an orgasm—helps retain more active sperm.[115] The message is clear: If you want to increase your chances of conceiving, relax and enjoy sex more.

Don't Get Hung Up on Timetable Sex

One great discovery that should help ease the pressure is that although making love in the week before and at the time of ovulation may help increase your chances of conception, the latest research has suggested that it may not be quite as important as previously thought.[e] A study conducted by the U.S. National Institute of Environmental Health Sciences (NIEHS) in North Carolina suggested that fertility-day timing is far less predictable than experts had thought, which will come as a great relief to women with irregular cycles who have no idea when they ovulate. Gynecologists have always known that ovulation day can vary a little, even for women with super-regular cycles, but they never realized how often this happened and to what extent. Now, the NIEHS figures suggest the possibility that even in healthy women with no fertility problems, ovulation isn't an exact science and may only occur around day 14 in one in three women.

This has caused quite a stir among fertility experts—but where does it leave a woman with PCOS? Learning to read your ovulation signals might help (see page 29), but even this has now been thrown into doubt by Canadian scientists whose research was published in July 2003 in the medical journal *Fertility and Sterility*. The Canadian study suggests that women experience far more hormonal surges each month than previously believed, and that each surge has the potential to produce an egg. If this is true, it will overturn 50 years of medical orthodoxy about the importance of timing in sex.

So now that there doesn't seem to be a better time for sex whether you have irregular or regular cycles, the best advice is probably the oldest: To maximize your chances of pregnancy, have as much intercourse as possible. Lots of sex will help normalize your cycles and help your partner, too, as the idea that abstaining from sex for up to a week so he can save up sperm isn't helpful. Abstaining will retain larger volumes of sperm, but at the same time, it will reduce the quality of the sperm; and poorer-quality sperm are less likely to make you pregnant, no matter how many of them there are.

Also, don't just have sex at night. Fertility experts believe that the most likely time for a woman to ovulate is at 4 P.M. If you can find somewhere private to meet, an excellent time to make love would be lunchtime—it would certainly brighten up your day!

So, you don't need to get obsessed with the idea of timetable sex. In fact, your body may very well help you feel more sexy at the right times anyway, with some researchers believing that, like many animals, a desire for mating in humans is when a female ovulates. Many women say that not only do they feel more sexy, but their partners feel more sexually stimulated when their wives or girlfriends are ovulating. So let nature take its course and have sex when you want to. You're more likely to enjoy it then, and this can also have fertility benefits.

The Importance of Orgasm

Although a man usually needs to have an orgasm for conception to happen, it's not necessary for a woman to have one. But it can help if the woman can climax after the man because the contractions of her womb and vagina create a partial vacuum, which will help to transport the sperm into her cervix. Without orgasm, they'll still get there, just not as quickly.

Research suggests that orgasm is a sophisticated way for women to unconsciously select which of her lovers' sperm is used to increase the chances of conception.[116] Two British biologists, Robin Baker and Mark Bellis, discovered that when a woman climaxes anytime between a minute before to 45 minutes after her lover ejaculates, she retains significantly more sperm than she does after nonorgasmic sex. In addition, their research results indicated that the strong muscular contractions associated with orgasm pull sperm from the vagina to the cervix, where it's in a better position to reach an egg. So it appears that on a physiological level, orgasm in women serves to favor the man she feels would make the best father for her child.

Satisfying Sex

Research also shows that women who have regular, satisfying sex, with intercourse at least once a week, have more regular menstrual cycles and fewer fertility problems than those who don't.[117] In addition, a satisfying sex life can be a wonderful way to reduce stress and therefore encourage fertility. How? In much the same way as exercise reduces the body's tension, which can interfere with hormone production, so can sex. The tension-releasing power of orgasm can be so great for some people that its effects are more powerful than a tranquilizer.

A loving, caring, emotionally supportive relationship can also have a positive effect on your fertility. Women can spontaneously ovulate when they fall in love, and there's growing evidence that when you feel happy, secure, and loved and have a fulfilling sex life, fertility can result. This isn't to say that being single or having an argument or breakup will affect your fertility, or that a bad relationship can't produce a baby, but if your love life is chronically stressful, it may contribute to your fertility problems.

Does It Matter Who's on Top?

With all this good news about how regular, enjoyable sex is the best way to boost fertility, why not turn that into an opportunity to experiment with a few positions to increase the fertility levels even more?

Are there ways you can make love to help you conceive? Yes, says fertility expert Dr. Niels Lauersen, an obstetrician/gynecologist with the St. Vincent Medical Center in New York City. He believes that "the positions both you and your partner assume during and right after making love can significantly affect the passage of sperm into your vagina to your fallopian tube."

Many experts believe that the man-on-top position has the best chance of getting a woman pregnant, but there are no studies to prove this. The rationale is that this position allows for deep penetration so the man's sperm can be ejaculated as close to the cervix as possible. This gives the sperm cells a good start on their long journey, as the closer they are to the ripe egg waiting in the fallopian tube a few inches farther up in a woman's body, the more likely they are to reach it.

Logically, any position that goes against gravity, such as the woman on top or having sex sitting or standing up, discourages the sperm's journey upward and is thought to deter conception.

If a man enters a woman from behind, especially if she's kneeling in front of him so she's at an angle with her bottom higher than her head, it's said to encourage conception. Making love in the "spoons" position (both partners facing the same way with the man penetrating the woman from behind) isn't thought to be such an effective baby-making position because the penetration angle isn't as deep. The chances might be maximized if the woman leaned the upper half of her body a little away from her partner, pushing her bottom against him.

Studies show that the best and fittest sperm have reached the fallopian tube in 5 minutes, and the rest usually get there within 45 minutes.[118] So as long as you don't leap up or go to the bathroom the moment you're finished, you probably don't need to be stuck on the floor or bed with one eye on the clock. In any case, it's the fastest and fittest sperm that you want to fertilize the egg.

In the words of Dr. Steven Brody of the Advanced Fertility Institute in San Diego, "The sperm that get in there right away have the best chance of fertilizing the egg. A study in rabbits shows that if you destroy all sperm in the vagina within five minutes, the rabbit can still get pregnant."

No Sex, Please—I'm Tired

It's all very well to know that you should be having regular sex in all sorts of fun positions, but what if you're too stressed and tired? Dr. Rosalind Bramwell, a fertility researcher at the University of Liverpool, says that "not being interested anymore is something that many couples don't like to admit to. Even to themselves."

A new condition called TINS (or "Two Incomes No Sex") is a real threat to fertility rates. More than half the people they interviewed said that their sex lives were suffering because of the long hours they spent at work, which meant that they felt too tired at the end of the day. Long hours are stressful, and sustained stress is also a well-recognized cause of clinical depression—and depression is the enemy of fertility in men and women.

If you're stressed and/or depressed, you may experience a wide range of symptoms, including fatigue and loss of appetite and libido. Should this be the case, it really is time to stop and take stock of the situation and think about what you need from the different areas of your life—and perhaps to talk it over with someone you trust, be it a friend, partner, doctor, or counselor. This can help clarify your thoughts and give you some support.

I'm Not in the Mood

"I really want to start a family with my partner, but we haven't had sex for about a year now. I really feel sorry for him, and he has a lot to put up with, but when I'm gaining weight, losing hair, getting pimples, and feeling unattractive because of PCOS, the last thing on my mind is sex. I'm just never in the mood." — Anna, 30 years old

If you never seem to feel in the mood for sex, and your libido is low, you aren't in the minority. In the February 1999 issue of *The Journal of the American Medical Association,* an astonishing report on the sexual health of Americans revealed that 43 percent of American women suffer from sexual dysfunction and loss of libido. The authors of the study noted that the "experience of sexual dysfunction is more likely among women with poor physical and emotional health and overall well-being." Poor health and lifestyle impair sexual drive and desire.

You may wonder why this is important. Well, the answer is threefold: First, whether you have PCOS or not, if you're in a relationship, lack of sexual desire is upsetting and likely to leave your mate feeling confused, embarrassed, or inadequate. Second, whether you have PCOS or not, if you don't have a fulfilling sex life, you're missing out on one of life's great pleasures. And third—again whether you have PCOS or not—sex is good for your health.

Sex Keeps You Young

Dr. David Weeks, clinical neuropsychologist at the Jardine Clinic of the Royal Edinburgh Hospital in Scotland, has studied thousands of people aged 18 to 102 who looked younger than their years. He concluded that they had up to 50 percent more sex than the national average (which, according to last year's Durex report, is 110 times a year), plus the women had more orgasms. "We think this is because when we feel pleasure, including sexual pleasure, our bodies release feel-good hormones called endorphins and human growth hormone—both of which slow the aging process, boost immunity, ease pain, and relieve stress. Sex can also boost your self-esteem and confidence, which helps you feel more positive about yourself and your life."

Yes, it's true that PCOS can make it more difficult for you to feel sexy, but it's important to understand that PCOS alone probably isn't the reason for loss of libido. For one, the hormone imbalance in PCOS isn't necessarily to blame, since raised testosterone should, in theory, increase your sex drive (testosterone therapy is becoming much more common as a libido-booster for menopausal women). So what's going on? As well as the possibility of poor physical and emotional health, if you aren't getting enough nutrients in your diet or exercising enough—or if you're feeling depressed—libido is one of the first things to suffer. But as we've seen in the fertility-boosting plan, there are steps you can take to improve your physical and emotional health. And by taking these steps toward a healthier you, the chances are your libido will improve, too.

It can take a month or two to really feel the benefits of the fertility boosting, so here are some reminders and ideas in the meantime.

Give Your Sex Life a Kick-Start

— Do eat healthfully according to the guidelines in our plan. Vitamins A and B, zinc, and selenium are all crucial for libido, and exercise also helps by boosting your mood and body image.

— Check your stress levels. "In general, stress dampens libido. A stressed woman may blame a host of other factors for her symptoms, without realizing that stress is the real cause of the problem," says Milwau.k.ee urologist and sex therapist Dr. Stuart Fine. (Deal with commonplace stress by following the de-stressing tips on page 33.)

— Depression is another major inhibitor of sexual desire. Try to understand why you're feeling low so that you can act appropriately when those times come again. If you feel that you can't cope alone, reach out for the support of family and friends, or see your doctor for referral to a counselor or therapist.

— Most sex therapists agree that sex begins in the head—in a way, it's an idea that overtakes you, and then your body's physical reaction follows. A key part of starting that sexual idea is setting the mood, and romantic music can help, as can low lighting, a candlelit bath, or your favorite romantic film. If you haven't felt sexy for a while, touching yourself can also be a way to reconnect with your body as a sensual, sexual pleasure. Once you're aware of your own desires again, it can be easier and less daunting to connect with your partner's.

— Reevaluate how you feel about your body. Remind yourself that your ability to become aroused, achieve sexual satisfaction, and reciprocate is there no matter what you weigh or look like. Stop focusing on what society tells you is beautiful, and concentrate instead on what you find beautiful and pleasurable about yourself.

— Relationship troubles can also contribute to loss of sexual desire. If you don't feel listened to, respected, or important, it's natural to respond with resentment, and that can dampen libido. It's important to open the lines of communication with your partner so that anger can be expressed in places other than the bedroom. If the source of the problem is severe, such as infidelity, you may want to go to a relationship counselor.

— If you find the idea of sex unappealing or uncomfortable, talk to a sex therapist to discuss your health, your upbringing, your circumstances, any body image issues you may have, and your relationship so that you can find ways to give yourself permission to satisfy your sexual needs. You may want to do this alone, or you may find that it's more productive to talk to a sex therapist with your partner.

— Make time for romance. Give it a higher priority in your life. However busy or stressful your life gets, try to make sure that you have some "couple time" where you can unwind together and talk about your day. And plan regular meals out, trips to the movies, or weekend breaks so that the two of you get some special time together away from the hustle and bustle of your daily life.

— Nature provides many safe, natural ways to boost sexual desire. Certain foods, such as chocolate, figs, and ginger, are thought to have aphrodisiac qualities because they contain nutrients that are essential for boosting libido, and any food that contains zinc, such as nuts or oysters, can be considered an aphrodisiac, since zinc is thought to have a positive effect on libido.

— There are numerous herbal treatments that are believed to help put sexual desire and drive back into your life. These include agnus castus, celery, wild oats, parsley, and damiana. If you want to take herbs to boost your libido, make sure you talk to a medical herbalist familiar with PCOS before self-prescribing.

— Aromatherapists suggest that certain scents can have an aphrodisiac effect. Michelle Roques-O'Neil produces a passion blend, containing jasmine, rose, patchouli, and sandalwood (see Resource Guide for details). This uplifting and sensual blend can be used in the bath, as a massage oil, or dabbed on your pulse points. Smell also works through association, so returning to a perfume you used to wear at the beginning of your relationship may rekindle the passion.

— Massage can help relax and invigorate as well. Treat yourself or your partner to a massage. California-based Robert Tisserand, founder of Tisserand Aromatherapy, suggests a sensual massage with the following oils: 30 drops of sweet-almond oil, 5 drops of ylang-ylang, 4 drops of lavender, and 3 drops of jasmine.

Keep Your Cool

You've probably heard stories of couples who tried really hard to get pregnant and only conceived when they gave up. Hence the notion of "trying too hard" that continues to be perpetuated. This may be true, but only when trying goes from being a natural, loving desire to have a baby into a demand filled with anxiety, fear, and worry, which are the real culprits.

Feel calm and confident about your sexuality and your ability to become a mother. Whether you have PCOS or not, maintaining the right emotional state is perhaps one of the best ways to enjoy your sex life and achieve conception. Make healthy diet and lifestyle choices, as our plan suggests, but above all . . . relax, stay calm, make love . . . and enjoy.

That's the Last Step . . . What Next?

The seven-step plan is a lot to take in all at once—so don't expect to be able to make the changes overnight. Ideally, you should be putting it in place over three or four months in order to give yourself and your partner a chance to get into the habit of following these guidelines so that they just become second nature. This isn't a "miracle" cure that will make you pregnant overnight—but you'll be amazed by how many women with PCOS have reported positive improvements in their symptoms and have gotten pregnant after getting their diets, emotions, and lifestyles into shape. So take a deep breath, be patient, and stick to the plan—you might be surprised by how dramatic the results are.

However, if you've been following the plan and you still have some problems to iron out—from irregular periods to unexplained nonconception—then it's time to move on to our fine-tuning section to tackle those issues.

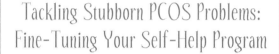

Chapter Three

Tackling Stubborn PCOS Problems: Fine-Tuning Your Self-Help Program

So you've been following the seven-step plan in the previous chapter of this book, and you're still having some problems. Well, whether you just want to get your body into its best shape for a possible pregnancy sometime in the future, or whether you've been trying for a while and the long-awaited pregnancy hasn't happened yet, it's time to look for some more solutions. Don't give up the seven steps, though—they're your basic foundation plan for boosting your fertility, and the advice in this section is designed to be used in addition to those steps to give you the added boost you need to conceive.

The general advice given to couples considering a pregnancy is to try for a year or two, and to see their doctor again if nothing's happened by the end of that time; but if you have PCOS, waiting any more than six months is bad advice—and if it comes from your doctor, find another one.

"If you have PCOS, think you have PCOS, or have irregular periods, don't wait a year to have the diagnosis of infertility. Seek help earlier," urges PCOS expert Dr. Samuel Thatcher. This is especially true if you're 35 or older, the age when fertility naturally starts to decline.

So now is the time to see your doctor for a health checkup. Getting a thorough examination for you and your partner—to determine sperm counts and check for blocked fallopian tubes or infections—is a really good thing to do. You may as well get all this worked out now so you know that you're going forward with every possible chance of maximizing your fertility.

Getting Your Partner's Fertility Checked

When asking for fertility treatment, your doctor or fertility specialist will ask for your partner's sperm to be checked, too. If the sperm is abnormal, he may be referred to an urologist or an andrologist, but a reproductive endocrinologist would be the best person to explain options and coordinate efforts. A question you should always ask when selecting a clinic is whether or not the team includes these specialists.

Don't be surprised if your partner gets anxious when asked for a semen sample at a fertility clinic. For a man to be told he has abnormal or poorly performing sperm is equivalent to a women being told she cannot carry a child. Men equate sperm counts with virility and manliness, and infertility can attack the male self-image as strongly as that of the female. And, as Dr. Thatcher states, "Women with PCOS often share lifestyle evils with their partners, and there is no better way than to work on the problems together." As we saw in the previous chapter, there's a close link between male obesity and decreased testosterone. Smoking, caffeine, and poor diet can affect sperm count, as can alcohol and certain medications. There's also the theory that increased heat can reduce sperm count. Without a doubt, research suggests that diet and lifestyle changes can have a positive effect.

———•———

If you and your partner have been given a clean bill of health, and if you and your doctor have identified that PCOS is definitely the problem, you can use the following self-help strategies to help overcome your particular issues, from irregular periods to being overweight; or you can use these techniques alongside fertility treatment, if this is the course of action you and your health-care provider decide is right. Taking these extra steps in addition to your basic fertility-boosting lifestyle plan will increase your chances of success when trying a conventional fertility program. Select the problem you want to focus on and use our advice to crank up your fertility another notch.

Stubborn Problem One: Irregular Periods

"I don't think I've ever had a regular menstrual cycle. It didn't used to worry me, but now that I'm thinking of starting a family, it does. I only have a period two or three times a year, and I'm worried about my fertility." — Rebecca, 30 years old

"My periods are in chaos. I really have no idea when—or if—I'm going to have one. Sometimes I cycle regularly, but then months will pass and nothing happens. I don't feel ill or tired, but somehow I don't feel right." — Sarah, 34 years old

"I'm 26, and I've never had a period. It was horrible at school when all my friends started. When I got to be 14 and nothing happened, I just pretended I had it—and I even went so far as to wear sanitary pads in P.E. lessons so they wouldn't suspect I was lying." — Mary, 26 years old

For most women with PCOS who are concerned about their fertility, irregular periods are probably the most common problem, and for good reason.[119] "The main issue is the regularity of a woman's cycle," says PCOS expert Dr. Adam Balen. "The less regular, the greater reduction in fertility."

Regular cycles are usually 23 to 35 days apart. But as long as your periods occur at roughly the same time each cycle—for example, they could be 45 days apart instead of the typical 28, but they always appear around day 45—they're classified as being regular. "In reality," says Toni Weschler, fertility awareness counselor and author of *Taking Charge of Your Fertility*, "cycles vary tremendously among women and often within each woman herself." This is because our bodies are affected by so many things, from diet to stress and medication.

If your periods are regular and your cycle length is less than 35 days, the odds are greater than 95 percent that you're ovulating, according to Dr. Balen. (This, of course, isn't the case if you're on the Pill. The Pill suppresses ovulation, and the periods you have when you're on it don't signify regular ovulation.) If there are long gaps between your periods, followed by a heavy one, this could mean that you aren't ovulating, as lack of ovulation is a common cause of heavy bleeding.

What Are Irregular Periods?

"If you have irregular periods, you simply don't know when your period is going to come," says Dr. Helen Mason. "You have no idea when and if you're ovulating—even a slightly irregular cycle means that timing intercourse is harder." The following symptoms are typical:

- Long stretches of time with no periods

- Some time without them, and then periods coming too quickly or bleeding continually for a few weeks

- Spotting between cycles

This can be disconcerting. As 34-year-old Linda says, "It's a weird feeling, kind of like when you need to sneeze but can't. I can't explain, but it just doesn't feel right." But there's no need to worry about backed-up flow, or the idea that there's a buildup of blood in your body because it isn't being shed every month.

"Rest assured that lack of menstruation doesn't result in an accumulation of toxins in your body," says Dr. Geoffrey Redmond, professor of pediatric endocrinology at The New York Hospital Cornell Medical Center. *Amenorrhea,* the medical term given to absent periods, doesn't involve the retention of menstrual fluid, because the menstrual fluid isn't being formed at all.

So how does this interfere with fertility? After all, you don't have periods when you're pregnant! The problem is that your womb usually only sheds its lining if ovulation has taken place during the cycle. Your period is actually triggered by an egg being released, as its empty follicle then pumps out progesterone in the second half of your cycle, and this eventually reaches a level that causes your uterine lining to shed as a period. So if you're not having a period, chances are you're not ovulating, and that's the reason you're not getting pregnant.

What Can You Do about It?

First, you need to look beyond your PCOS for a moment. Although irregular periods are a common symptom of the disease, they're also caused by lots of other day-to-day things, and you need to rule those out before you focus all your energy on fine-tuning your PCOS self-care program.

Crash dieting, stress, seasonal changes, travel (especially long-distance airplane flights), heavy exercise, and illness can all cause a disruption in your cycle, and periods usually return when full health is recovered and stress is reduced.[120] For example, as we explained in the previous chapter, if you don't have enough fat because of dieting, exercise, or other weight loss, your body will think that you're starving. Since it's not appropriate to get pregnant when food is scarce, research has shown that your body will simply shut down your menstrual cycle. Periods will stop or become irregular until you get some fat back.[121]

In a similar way, when it's under stress, your body reacts to the crisis by affecting your menstrual cycle—which is nature's way of protecting you from pregnancy when it's less likely that you'll cope. It's well known that women going through a bereavement or any other kind of major trauma can stop menstruating. "You can't fool your body," says Sarah Berga, M.D., associate professor of obstetrics, gynecology, and psychiatry at the University of Pittsburgh. "Your body knows. It makes a judgment call. It knows that it is under stress, and since it won't have enough energy to maintain vital functioning, it gets rid of the reproductive cycle until health has been restored."

The occasional skipped or late period isn't anything to panic about, but it *is* a warning sign. Your body is trying to tell you that you're not 100 percent well. But if you've had irregularities for more than three cycles, or if your periods have simply stopped altogether, the likely cause isn't stress or an upset in your routine, but PCOS, according to Dr. James Douglas, reproductive endocrinologist from the Plano Medical Center in Texas. (Do bear in mind, however, that other conditions, such as fibroids, thyroid disorders, infection, eating disorders, and chronic illness, can all cause menstrual irregularity. If you have any of these, or suspect that they could be playing a part, ask your doctor to rule them out.)

Why Does PCOS Cause Irregular Periods?

As we explained in the first chapter, the menstrual cycle in women with PCOS is often irregular because they can't have a period without ovulation—and in some of these women, the eggs aren't being developed and released due to the imbalance of hormones in the body.

It seems that in women with PCOS, follicles start to mature, but for some reason they fail to ripen properly or to be released. Instead, they stay in the ovaries and continue to produce estrogen, but no progesterone. Remember, progesterone is the hormone that prepares your body for pregnancy if an egg is fertilized by a sperm, or for menstruation if no egg is fertilized. Over time, more and more empty egg follicles build up so that the ovaries become filled with these "cysts," as they're called, and with hard fibrotic growths that show up on an ultrasound screen.

This pattern could continue for many months, and for some women with PCOS, it does—they can go for 2 to 24 months or more without a period. For other women, the lining of the womb, which has become overgrown due to estrogen production, begins to break down of its own accord, and they experience spotting or heavy bleeding. In some cases, a follicle does eventually manage to develop, ovulation occurs, and a new cycle begins.

"Unfortunately, there are still no clear answers as to why this happens," says Dr. Douglas. "All we do know is that there are problems in the hormonal-feedback loop that regulates the menstrual cycle." Elevated levels of luteinizing hormone (LH) and estrogen have been found in some, but not all, women with PCOS, and this can block ovulation.[122] Research by Stephen Franks, professor of reproductive endocrinology at Imperial College, London, has shown that higher than normal levels of the hormone testosterone are also associated with PCOS and irregular periods (testosterone inhibits ovulation).[123] Research has also focused on why some women with PCOS have higher than normal levels of insulin.[124-5] It's possible that elevated levels of insulin encourage testosterone production by the ovaries and contribute to menstrual disturbances, but the general consensus is that inappropriate levels of LH, estrogen, insulin, and testosterone are, again, symptoms rather than causes of PCOS. The root cause or causes remain unknown at this time.

So, How Can I Tell If I'm Ovulating?

It's possible to have periods and not ovulate, but regular periods are generally a good indication that you're ovulating—even if you only have four or five periods a year. Yet if they're irregular, chances are you aren't ovulating (also see page 29 in Chapter 2).

Ovulation-Predictor Kits

You might be tempted to buy ovulation-predictor kits from your pharmacist. These contain a simple dipstick urine test that you can do at home. They work by detecting the surge of LH that happens 24–36 hours before ovulation. However, women with PCOS often have higher than normal levels of LH, so it wouldn't be wise to rely on these at-home tests, because you may get inaccurate results. Also, if your periods are irregular, you can never be sure when ovulation occurs, so you could end up buying lots of kits and wasting a lot of money.

"Your body gives you conspicuous signs," says Toni Weschler, "to help you understand on a daily basis what is transpiring within." Certain key signals occur to suggest that ovulation—and your peak fertility time—are near, and it's probably better for women with PCOS to learn how to read these signs, rather than relying on the tests described above.

The fertile-mucus sign is the most important indicator, as you may find that you don't experience any of the others. So what is fertile mucus? It's clear, watery, and stretchy, like the white of runny egg. The most important fertility signal of all, it's also the easiest to detect. (*Note:* If you have a vaginal infection, you may not be able to detect fertility signals.) Other signs include:

1. **Feeling sexier:** Some women say that they're more interested in sex around this time.

2. **Ovulation pain:** There may be a dull ache or twinge on one side of the abdomen, low down, that lasts for a few moments or a whole day.

3. **Softer cervix:** It will feel less firm and softer than usual when you touch it gently with your finger.

4. **Spotting:** A tiny loss of blood can sometimes occur at ovulation. If you notice it, talk to your doctor and make sure that your cervix is healthy before linking this to ovulation.

5. **Temperature:** Body temperature drops slightly before ovulation and increases by about 0.4°F afterward. Temperature checking can seem quite complicated, and it usually takes a few months to get the hang of it, so it may be best to see a natural-family-planning counselor who can help you learn this method.

What Choices Do I Have Now?

In order for you to have a normal menstrual cycle where ovulation does occur, you need to get your hormones back in balance. Your doctor will probably suggest the Pill or an insulin-sensitizing drug called *metformin* (see the Glossary for more information) to regulate your periods, but neither of these get to the root of the problem, the real reason *why* your periods are irregular. For example, the Pill will regulate your cycle, but you won't actually be having real periods. What you're getting instead is caused by withdrawal from the effects of the Pill, so when you stop taking this contraception, symptoms it suppressed are likely to return, and you certainly can't get pregnant if you're on it.

The insulin-sensitizing effects of metformin don't correct the diet and lifestyle factors that may be contributing to blood-sugar imbalances, but it can trigger ovulation and regular periods by causing weight loss. "Just be aware that metformin is not a magic bullet," says Gerard Conway, a consultant gynecologist at Middlesex Hospital, London. "It won't work long term if diet and exercise plans are not in place."

You can also encourage hormonal balance, and therefore a more regular cycle, with the following self-care strategies.

1. **Improve your diet**, using the guidelines outlined in the seven-step fertility-boosting plan in Chapter 2. We can't stress enough how many women have written to us after using our PCOS diet book to say that it's helped them regain their health, especially by restoring lost periods. Healthy eating can seem like a chore, but don't worry—if you manage to stick to the rules 80 percent of the time, you're doing really well. If you're still finding that your periods are unpredictable, try these extra few steps to kick-start them, as research shows that blood sugar– and hormone-balancing dietary approaches can really help.[126-7]

— *Keep your blood sugar balanced* by eating the right carbs (complex, low glycemic index (GI) foods, such as vegetables, whole-grain bread, basmati rice, and legumes), cutting down on sugar, and eliminating products made with refined white flour. This ensures healthy insulin and blood-sugar levels, and also helps you feel fuller for longer, which prevents overeating. Always eat breakfast and have small, frequent meals throughout the day (or three main meals and two healthy snacks), no more than three hours apart to avoid rapid fluctuations in blood sugar. Eat a little protein and fiber with each meal to slow down your body's release of sugar into your bloodstream and keep your insulin levels stable.

— A new study led by PCOS expert Dr. Adam Balen, to be published in 2004 or 2005, suggests that *a low-GI diet* can help control the symptoms of PCOS, and that many women with this syndrome have reported weight-loss success when eating foods that have a low glycemic index. The glycemic index is a guideline for diabetics that measures the impact a food has on blood sugar when eaten. Foods with high values (such as sugar, bananas, white bread, and corn chips) should be avoided in favor of low-GI foods (such as legumes, beans, apples, and oatmeal). To find out more, ask your doctor for a list of the GI values of different foods.

— *Phytoestrogens* have been shown to have a balancing effect on hormones and periods.[128] Found in all fruits, vegetables, and grains, they're most beneficial in the form of isoflavones, which are found in garlic and in legumes such as soybeans, lentils, beans, and chickpeas. These foods have a mild estrogenic effect and can help balance estrogen levels because their phytoestrogen molecules bond to the body's own estrogen receptors. The phytoestrogens are only weak in comparison to the body's own estrogens, so they can help where there is excess estrogen, as in anovulatory (no ovulation) PCOS; or when an estrogen boost is needed—after menopause, for example. Phytoestrogens also have been found to stimulate the production of sex hormone-binding globulin (SHBG). SHBG is a protein produced by the liver that binds sex hormones like estrogen in order to control how many of them are circulating in your blood. Having the right amount of SHBG gives you a better chance of hormone balance.[129]

The phytochemical DIM (Indole-3-Carbinol or IC3), found in cruciferous vegetables, may also have a beneficial effect on your cycle by helping regulate estrogen, but because it isn't helpful if your testosterone levels are high, more research needs to be done to see if it's a suitable treatment for women with PCOS.[130]

How Much Soy?

Soy hasn't had very good press in the last few years: It's been linked to thyroid problems, mineral deficiencies, and birth defects. In reality, most of these concerns have little scientific backing and have been conducted on animals rather than humans. There's no denying that soy can block the uptake of certain nutrients that are essential for thyroid function, but this is only when eaten raw and in excess.

In moderation, soy is good for you and your fertility—so do eat it, as it can have a dramatic effect on your hormones, your health, and your well-being. But don't go overboard. Include it in your diet three to five times a week, not every day, and eat it in its natural form, avoiding supplements and choosing products such as miso, tofu, or organic soy milk.

— *Make sure you're avoiding saturated fats* from most animal and full-fat dairy products by choosing skim varieties, cutting the fat off your meat, or using low-fat cooking methods such as grilling. We recommend this because saturated fats block your body's absorption of essential fatty acids (EFAs) and stimulate estrogen production, which isn't helpful if you have irregular periods.[131]

But don't cut fat out altogether: Some is essential for every cell in your body and is crucial to help regulate your periods by balancing your hormones. The U.K. Department of Health suggests that we should double our intake of omega-3 EFAs by eating oily fish two or three times a week. Other sources of omega-3 include nuts, seeds, or flaxseed oil; and, to some extent, pumpkin seeds, walnuts, and dark green veggies. Research has shown that women taking 10 g (0.35 oz.) of ground flaxseed per day increase the regularity of their cycles and improve ovulation.[132] Flaxseeds also have a phytoestrogenic effect, so eat them sprinkled on cereal, baked in bread, added to salads or soups, or just as a teaspoon-a-day supplement.

— *Use proven nutritional supplements,* but remember that they aren't a substitute for a healthy diet. Ideally, you should see a nutritionist or dietitian for a personalized recommendation. "Eating healthily and gently detoxing your diet are the priority if you have irregular periods and PCOS," says nutrition expert Dr. Adam Carey. "Supplements should be seen as a way to support these positive changes. A nutritionist would typically prescribe a good multivitamin and mineral, along with an antioxidant complex and essential fatty acid supplement for women with PCOS and irregular periods."

If you're not already doing so, start taking a good multivitamin and mineral every day. It should contain the recommended daily amounts (RDA) of vitamin B6 (which improves ovulation rates, resulting in pregnancy), magnesium (since a deficiency is tied to irregular cycles),[133-4] and 30 mg of zinc (a crucial mineral for your menstrual cycle and fertility).

You may also want to boost your healthy diet further with a good antioxidant formula and essential fatty acids (good amounts of omega-3 and omega-6 essential oils), which have been proven to help regulate the cycle. Dosage guidance from nutritionist Marilyn Glenville specifies supplementing with 150 g of omega-6 and at least 2 g of omega-3 each day. (See pages 39–42 in Chapter 2 for more on vitamins and minerals.)

2. **Keep sugar cravings at bay.** Do you find it difficult to stay away from sugary snacks? You'll really improve your health and fertility by cutting down, so begin the process by identifying your triggers. Are there certain places, such as supermarkets or parties; or certain emotions, such as fear and anger; or certain activities, such as watching TV, that make you reach for a chocolate bar? The more you become aware of your triggers, the more you can start to deal with them. When the craving starts, try doing something else instead, such as taking a walk or doing some gardening.

If you get the urge to eat, ride it out. Food cravings peak and subside like waves, so when you get the desire for sugar, tell yourself that you can satisfy it if you need to—then wait a few moments, which will allow most cravings time to subside. As we recommended above, if just waiting is too difficult, try doing something to distract yourself.

Here are some more ideas to help cut down on unhealthy eating:

— *Don't go shopping when you're hungry* because you'll end up buying sugary snacks.

— *Stock up on healthy snacks*—fruit with a handful of nuts, low-fat crackers with low-fat cottage cheese, or bite-sized vegetables such as baby carrots—and have them close at hand or in your refrigerator for when temptation strikes.

— *Explore your local health-food store.* Rice cakes with bananas, pure fruit spread, or peanut butter make delicious snacks.

— *When you want comfort food, make yourself hot chocolate* with skim or soy milk, or some oatmeal with honey.

— *Smelling vanilla essential oil can prevent cravings for sweet foods,* according to research from St. George's Hospital in London. Drop some oil on a tissue and inhale when you feel the need.[135–6]

3. Take extra care of your liver. If you're following the detox guidelines in the seven-step plan, you're already ahead in terms of detoxing, But to end irregular periods, it may be worth giving your liver some extra pampering. Your liver processes harmful toxins, waste products, and hormones. For example, it deals with surplus estrogen so that it can be eliminated from your body. If this organ isn't functioning well, old hormones remaining after each menstrual cycle can accumulate—and if they're not deactivated by the liver, they can return to the bloodstream and cause trouble. Make sure that you eliminate any substances that can compromise your liver, especially alcohol. You may also want to supplement with B vitamins because they're essential for your liver to process estrogen (the herb milk thistle is also excellent, as studies have shown that it can increase the number of new liver cells to replace old, worn-out ones).[137]

Stubborn Problem Two: Needing to Lose Some Weight

As we saw in the fertility-boosting plan, weight management is a key to good health and fertility if you have PCOS—but it's often one of the trickiest aspects to get right and can be very frustrating, as PCOS tends to make gaining easy and losing more difficult. As we stressed in the previous chapter, research has shown that this problem is four times more likely if you have PCOS and irregular periods than if you don't, yet research has shown that weight management can trigger ovulation and regular cycles in women who have stopped ovulating.[138-40]

Following the guidelines already discussed is a good start—and if you feel you need an extra boost, we have some more options for you.

Ditch Fad Diets!

"It's really unfair, but women with PCOS just don't seem to burn off calories as most people do," says Dr. Helen Mason, senior lecturer in reproductive endocrinology at St. George's Hospital Medical School in London. But don't be tempted by fad-driven diet plans that promise fast weight loss, since they won't help you—or your fertility—in the long run.

Crash dieting is the biggest no-no if you have PCOS, because it just puts your body into starvation mode and sends your insulin metabolism into an even worse state; and sudden weight loss can actually stop your periods, too.

What about those high-protein and low- or no-carbohydrate diets that are so popular these days? Two studies presented to the Endocrine Society meeting in San Francisco in June 2002 suggest that "low carbing" isn't helpful for long-term health if you have PCOS, as you end up eating high-fat, low-nutrient foods that don't give you the nutrients, fiber, or essential fats you need for hormonal well-being and a healthy heart. (You want to be around when your kid(s) grow up, after all!) Instead, it's cutting calories by replacing sugar and high-fat food with nutritious food and increasing activity levels that matters, as we stress with our advice in the seven-step fertility-boosting plan in the previous chapter. Don't throw out that sound, healthy eating advice if you're finding weight loss difficult—stick to protein with every meal and choose the right, low-GI carbs such as vegetables, legumes, and whole-grain bread and pasta as the basis for your eating plan.

— **Remember: A Few Pounds Could Be Enough!** If you're overweight, the good news is that to have a regular cycle you don't need to be stick thin. "Sometimes just losing a few pounds can make a big difference to the way you ovulate," says Professor Franks of Imperial College, London.

— **Don't Overdo the Exercise.** It's a must for optimal health and fertility, but taken to extremes, working out can cause periods to become irregular or even stop. Check with your doctor to see if your routine is appropriate.

Tackle Emotional Eating

"I find it hard to get by without chocolate and other sweets. I know they aren't good for me physically, and they probably make my symptoms worse, but they make me feel better emotionally. I've tried cutting down, but sometimes I feel so low that only a bar of chocolate will do." — Mandy, 24 years old

Losing weight can be a difficult issue, especially if you have PCOS. But if you're struggling to stick to a healthy eating regime in order to boost your fertility, it's time to look at your relationship with food. After all, until you sort this out, you're making it extra hard for yourself to adhere to any new diet plan.

So, do *you* comfort yourself with foods that you know aren't good for you? Many women have a complex relationship with food and eat in response to stress or difficult and painful emotions. With PCOS, the problem can intensify due to the moods swings and sugar cravings often linked with the condition; and then there are the body-image insecurities and weight-management problems that become a part of the big picture as well. So if you want to change to a healthy eating plan, it's crucial that you first heal your emotional relationship with food because you're setting yourself up for struggling and feelings of failure if you don't.

If you know that you always reach for the cake or chocolate when you're feeling blue or stressed, your first step to improved fertility through good nutrition isn't to focus on *what* you're eating, but to understand *why* you're eating it. This way, you can move toward a more healthy attitude and free yourself from emotional eating. Once you do so, you can eat what's good for you without feeling deprived and enjoy the occasional treat without feeling guilty. Whether you need to deal with stress or depression, get your mood swings under control, or build your self-esteem and body image, you need to stop these issues that are sabotaging your weight-loss plan. (To find the right support, information, and advice, see our Resource Guide.)

Get Medical Help

If weight loss is proving frustrating, and you know it could really help improve your chances of conception, you don't have to struggle alone. Talk to your doctor about getting a referral to a dietician or nutritionist who can work out a personalized plan and help you stick to it.

However, if you have a lot of weight to lose, there are more serious measures you can discuss with your doctor, such as drugs like *sibutramine* (sold under the brand name Meridia in the United States). Sibutramine is an appetite suppressant—basically, it makes you feel satisfied with less food. Women with PCOS can lose weight on this drug, but there can be unpleasant side effects, which include nausea, headaches, and an unpleasant taste in the mouth, and it isn't ideal if you aren't eating that much already. Most important, it also may not be safe if you're pregnant or actively trying to have a baby.

Another option is a new diet pill that's thought to be able to help people quit smoking and lose weight at the same time. This drug, *rimonabant,* works by blocking the circuits in the brain that control the urge to eat and smoke. The makers, the French firm Sanofi-Synthelabo, hope to market it in 2005 since it's shown promising results so far. In one trial, rimonabant helped people shed an average of 20 pounds in a year; in another, it was found to double the chances of smokers successfully quitting (at least in the short term). Dr. Robert Anthenelli of the University of Cincinnati, who directed the smoking study, said, "We think this might be the ideal compound for people who are overweight and smoke." However, it's important to point out that, like sibutramine, rimonabant may not be safe to take if you're pregnant or trying to be. As always, discuss all medications with your doctor.

Your health-care team can also look at ketosis, a method where you eat only high-protein foods to encourage your body to break down fat. This is still a controversial method for women with PCOS, as experts can't agree on whether it's safe in the long term, but in the short term, it can offer the benefits of fast weight loss for women who really need to lose a lot of weight. However, it must be done under medical supervision with regular monitoring.

Metformin (mentioned earlier on page 85) could also be an option. There have been several studies reporting good results with metformin for weight loss. Primarily a treatment for diabetes, it's become associated with PCOS because of its ability to decrease insulin resistance and the belief that it may improve fertility.

Stubborn Problem Three: A Stressed-Out Lifestyle

Sometimes it's easier to take on diet plans and exercise routines than it is to look at the stressed-out whirl your life has become. If it's been simpler for you to change your eating habits and how much you exercise than to unwind and reduce your feelings of stress (which can mount up when you're trying to have a baby, too), then you need to focus on this area for a while. It's amazing how many of the women with PCOS we talked to found that even when they were doing everything else right, this one piece of the puzzle wasn't fitting into place. But when it did, their periods came back, and pregnancy often followed.

> *"It's worth investing in de-stressing your life. I was so rigid in following a healthy diet and exercise plan, making sure I was doing well at work, staying in touch with my family and elderly parents, as well as trying to fit in romantic evenings with my husband in order to try to get in the mood for baby making, that I was wound up really tight. A friend of mine who didn't have*

PCOS, but who'd found it difficult to get pregnant, suggested that I start going for massages, having some chill-out time, and looking after myself instead of my career and my family for a change—and something just clicked. I started having massages, giving myself the time for long baths and reading books, and turning down invitations from friends and family just to have some time for me and for my marriage. Just four months later I got pregnant." — Naomi, 34 years old, who has a 3-year-old son

So how does stress have such a powerful effect on fertility, and why is it worth trying to reduce it if you have PCOS and are struggling to conceive?

If you're under stress, too much prolactin is released, and the normal messages between your brain (hypothalamus and pituitary) and ovaries can be affected, interfering with your ovaries' ability to produce the right balance of hormones.[141] The following techniques can help:

Invest in Some "Me" Time

If the ideas in the seven-step plan aren't helping you unwind, it's time to invest in a bigger commitment to time for yourself.

As we suggested in the previous chapter, studies have shown how yoga and meditation can help ease tension, but yoga can do far more than that. Studies have shown that the deep breathing and stretching exercises of yoga can also help restore hormonal balance.[142] Meditation can also stimulate feelings of calm and tranquility and enhance your feelings of control,[143] so try this mini meditation to get you started.

Mini Meditation

Find a place where you feel comfortable, and imagine each part of your body relaxing. Begin with your scalp and work down to your toes while mentally repeating a neutral thought (try a color or a cloudless sky). Concentrate on your breathing, and when thoughts break through the calm, which they will, just let them come and go. After five minutes, open your eyes and sit quietly for a few moments before getting up and continuing your day.

Home Aromatherapy

Aromatherapy is a natural treatment that uses the therapeutic properties of essential oils, extracted from the flowers, leaves, stem barks, or wood of aromatic plants and trees. Essential oils are extremely potent concentrates that can be absorbed through the skin or by inhaling, and are often used in massage and while bathing. Oils applied to the skin may affect you for several hours, while those that are inhaled will stimulate the limbic system in the brain, which deals with emotions.

Aromatherapist and reflexologist Frances Box, who works out of clinics in Surrey and Sussex in the U.K., says she chooses aromatherapy oils both to help regulate the hormonal imbalances that are causing menstrual irregularity, and also to aid relaxation and release stress, which can exacerbate this condition.

Aromatherapy Oils for Stress and Period Problems

Oils of particular relevance for helping soothe stress and restore irregular periods are lavender, clary sage, geranium, jasmine, melissa (lemon balm), rose, sandalwood, neroli, and ylang ylang.

Massage your abdomen, neck, and shoulders as often as possible (or get a friend or partner to do it for you so you can totally relax!), using a total of two drops of your chosen therapeutic oil mixed with a teaspoon of carrier oil, such as sweet-almond oil or pure sunflower oil. You can also soak in a warm bath treated with a total of four drops of essential oil, diluted by a teaspoon of carrier oil or a tablespoon of whole milk. Try unwinding to the scent of your favorite oil dropped onto a vaporizer or burner. Try to turn your aromatherapy treatment into a regular treat, and really enjoy it, safe in the knowledge that it's doing you a world of good.

If you've tried these techniques to beat your stubborn PCOS problems and you still feel that you need more help on your way to conception, the next chapters, which describe additional natural and medical fertility treatments, are for you. If you have the time and the inclination, you could try the natural therapies first, before moving on to medical intervention. On the other hand, you and your health-care provider may decide that it's best for you to use the natural alternatives at the same time as the conventional methods. Either way, you'll have the information you need.

Chapter Four

Fertility Treatment the Natural Way: Your Options with Complementary Therapies

As we've seen in the previous chapters, there's a lot you can do on your own to boost your fertility, but now we'll begin to look at what other people can do to help, too. If you feel it's the right time to try professional fertility treatments, natural complementary therapies have a lot to offer, as long as you choose a reputable, well-qualified practitioner. Meanwhile, continue your self-help program in order to enhance the power of any new programs because the healthier you are, the sooner they'll start working.

You may want to try this combination of self-help and complementary regimens for a few months or longer, depending on where you are in your journey. But you can also combine them with medical help (discussed in Chapter 5) for a triple treatment, if that feels right to you.

What Does Complementary Mean?

The term *complementary therapies* describes options that research tentatively shows can be used effectively to complement, or support, mainstream treatment.[144] Philip Holm, chairman of Issue, the national fertility association of the U.K., says, "Due to increased coverage in the media of the alternative field, people are more open to trying more holistic methods to boost their fertility. Many of our members have used alternative therapies and believe they have been successful."

Practitioners of alternative medicine also claim that they can help women with PCOS conceive, but medical experts still differ wildly in their opinions.[145] You'll need to discuss this with your health-care provider, ideally seeking their support if you want to try this route. Get several recommendations for a good complementary-therapy specialist who's happy to share information with you and your doctor so that you can all work together.

Current PCOS research can't give definitive statistics on what will work for whom and for how long, since so little has been done to explore this avenue: "It's a tricky one and more research is needed," says Dr. Simon Fishel, director of the Centers for Assisted Reproduction (CARE) at Park Hospital in Nottingham, U.K., "but I have an open mind. Fertility seems to be affected by so many factors—lifestyle, stress, emotions—and maybe alternative medicine is addressing these issues, so I do feel there is a place for it."

Now don't forget the fact that these are natural therapies, which means you can use them to assist, enhance, and support more conventional treatments. As women's-health and holistic-medicine specialist Dr. Sarah Temple (see the Resource Guide) says, "Complementary therapies are useful for rebalancing the body and making women feel ready for pregnancy. A lot of my patients have found acupuncture or reflexology helpful. If you do decide to have IVF [in vitro fertilization], it's stressful. These women were glad they were also doing hypnotherapy, meditation, or yoga to help them cope."

We're not saying that alternative therapies don't have physical effects, but until more research is done, we won't know in scientific or medical terms what those effects are. But within the PCOS community on the Internet, there's a growing feeling that many of these therapies do seem to work.

Be Careful in Your Choice

Having problems trying to get pregnant can make you very vulnerable, so you need to make sure that you aren't being cheated or deceived. "Always choose someone who has been registered with the appropriate training organization," says Nicky Wesson, author of *Alternative Infertility Treatments*. "Find a therapy which feels right for you. Do your research and make an informed decision of what you feel may work for you. Find a therapist you like and trust and avoid anything which your intuition tells you is extreme or inappropriate." She also suggests that you should be cautious about any therapist who expects you to spend hundreds of dollars on products that can only be bought from them.

Make sure that all your health-care providers communicate well with you and with each other, and that you've had a medical diagnosis (so that you know PCOS is definitely the problem). In addition, use as many e-mail groups, support groups, and other contacts as possible in order to find out which natural therapy and practitioner seems right for you. Here are some uplifting stories we heard while researching this book that might inspire you to explore these types of treatment:

> Sarah had been trying for four years to get pregnant. She was diagnosed with PCOS when she came off the Pill at age 24, and the consultant told her bluntly that without fertility treatment, it was unlikely she would get pregnant. After fertility drugs failed, IVF was suggested. *"I couldn't face it,"* she says. *"That night, I logged on to a PCOS Website where a woman recommended reflexology for infertility, so I made an appointment with a local practitioner for my lunch hour. The reflexologist explained that this therapy rebalances the body's energy by placing pressure on certain parts of the feet. She worked on the areas linked to reproduction, as well as the pituitary gland, which controls hormones, and told me to spend five minutes a night massaging below my anklebones to stimulate my ovaries. To my amazement, three months later I discovered I was*

pregnant. And my 20-week ultrasound showed it was twins. My reflexologist had worked a miracle after just ten sessions."

Sophie didn't start trying to have a baby until she was well into her 30s. After two years, she finally got pregnant at age 36. Then, at 14 weeks, the pain and bleeding began, and she miscarried. A year later she got pregnant again, but miscarried at eight weeks. *"I made repeated visits to my doctor,"* she says, *"but I was told that this was normal since I had PCOS, and fertility treatment wouldn't help—I simply had to keep trying. After my third miscarriage was followed by weeks of bleeding, I changed doctors, and by chance, my new physician was trained in homeopathy. She gave me sepia 30 for the bleeding. I'd never heard of homeopathy before and had no idea what it could do, but I took the tablets—and the bleeding stopped. She also gave me natrum muriaticum, which made me feel calmer immediately.*

"I was impressed: She treated me like an individual and helped me understand PCOS and not be frightened of it. When I got pregnant for the fourth time, I was determined that this one would succeed. My doctor advised me on what I should be eating and gave me homeopathic remedies to help. And finally, nine months later, I gave birth to a healthy baby girl. I was 39 years old and never thought I'd have a baby, but once I had the help of homeopathy, it happened without a hitch."

Paula was 33 when she was diagnosed with PCOS, and doctors suggested Clomid. *"Friends of mine had taken it and felt fine,"* she says, *"but I felt awful. My emotions went crazy—it felt like PMS times a thousand, and the moodiness was like nothing I'd experienced before. I didn't get pregnant, so I tried Clomid again and experienced the same horrendous side effects.*

"At that time, a friend of mine who was studying acupuncture needed volunteers to practice on, so I volunteered. After the first session, I was buzzing, and the awful moodiness Clomid had caused disappeared. I felt like me again. Mentally I felt different,

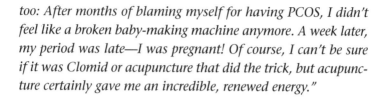

too: After months of blaming myself for having PCOS, I didn't feel like a broken baby-making machine anymore. A week later, my period was late—I was pregnant! Of course, I can't be sure if it was Clomid or acupuncture that did the trick, but acupuncture certainly gave me an incredible, renewed energy."

After four failed attempts at IVF, 40-year-old Katherine found an article on alternative therapists who'd helped women get pregnant and decided to try hypnotherapy. *"It was a tearful meeting at first,"* she says, *"because telling the hynotherapist everything that had happened made me realize how much I ached to have a baby, and how as each year went by, my chances were getting slimmer and slimmer. The ten-week course she suggested was all about unblocking the obstacles in my subconscious that could stop me from becoming pregnant without me being aware of them. I decided to give it a try.*

"At each session, I was put in a trancelike state. Counting down from ten to zero, the hynotherapist told me to imagine walking slowly down some stairs to a beautiful garden, and then she asked me about my life. One thing that we talked about a lot was how I'd felt when my periods started. I remembered feeling embarrassed and hiding it for nearly a year. When I finally told my mom, she gasped in horror and made me feel that 'the curse' was something to be ashamed of. But instead of hating my periods, the hypnotherapist said I should embrace them because they made me a woman. Visualizing myself as a mother with a healthy baby was also key to the treatment. Six months after the sessions, I was pregnant, and I gave birth to a healthy baby boy nine months later. Nothing has ever made me feel so happy."

Which Therapies Work Well with PCOS?

Most complementary therapies look at you as a whole person whose body, emotions, lifestyle, and experience all play a part in creating any health problems you're having. Since the main root of the

PCOS fertility problem is underlying metabolic and hormonal imbalances, therapists from most nontraditional disciplines will take a natural approach to creating hormonal harmony in order to facilitate regular periods, ovulation, and the right conditions in your body and mind to encourage conception.

The choices you make will depend on your particular condition, which therapy sounds appealing or seems logical, and recommendations from friends or other women with PCOS. Another good way to find a local, well-qualified practitioner is by contacting the associations governing national standards of practice and qualifications, who will list all their accredited practitioners for you (see the Resource Guide).

Although medical expert opinion is still divided, many women with PCOS we spoke to found that the natural therapies discussed in this chapter had profound results when administered by a properly qualified therapist, who ideally will have knowledge of PCOS or experience in treating PCOS patients. We chose these remedies because they're the ones we found that most women had used with positive results, and/or they have some research backing them up as valid options to explore. But remember: Always seek the help of a qualified practitioner before trying them, since some aren't recommended for use during pregnancy.

Nutritional Therapy Plus Lifestyle Changes

The ideas we've presented in the last few chapters are effective and can mostly be carried out on your own, but in addition to suggesting healthful eating and lifestyle changes, a nutritionist can help you figure out what specific nutrients you may be lacking, and then choose a diet and supplements uniquely tailored for you and your lifestyle.

Much of the advice given by a nutritionist will be the same as that given in the PCOS fertility-boosting action plan. You've seen how important preconceptual care is for increasing your chances of conceiving, and you've also seen how healthy lifestyle recommendations

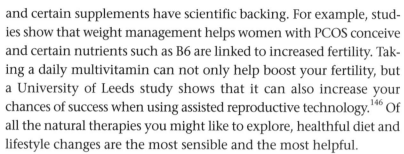
and certain supplements have scientific backing. For example, studies show that weight management helps women with PCOS conceive and certain nutrients such as B6 are linked to increased fertility. Taking a daily multivitamin can not only help boost your fertility, but a University of Leeds study shows that it can also increase your chances of success when using assisted reproductive technology.[146] Of all the natural therapies you might like to explore, healthful diet and lifestyle changes are the most sensible and the most helpful.

(*Note:* When taking any kind of supplement, always seek advice from a dietitian, doctor, or nutritionist before self-medicating.)

Herbal Medicine

Along with nutritional therapy, acupuncture, and reflexology, herbalism seems to be the most popular choice for women with PCOS, and it's had some very good results. Many women think it's logical to simply use the medicinal power of plants in their natural state to improve health and well-being, as opposed to using synthesized extracts or isolated compounds the way that many drugs do—and so many synthetic drugs are based on plants anyway. For instance, aspirin is extracted from white willow bark; the heart drug digitalis comes from foxglove; and the diabetes drug metformin that's now being used for PCOS was inspired by an herb called goat's rue.

"Western medical herbalism can be extremely effective in balancing the hormones, increasing the function of the ovaries, and improving the function of the pituitary gland (the master gland that controls the hormones in the body). Many women with irregular cycles have found that herbs are excellent for balancing their hormones and therefore regulating their cycles and aiding conception," says Julie Whitehouse, senior lecturer in medical herbs at the University of Westminster, London.

A medical herbalist, according to Whitehouse, will take your full medical and personal history and look at your lifestyle, diet, and environment. They'll ask about any vitamins, minerals, or drugs that you might be taking, and make any necessary recommendations. They then may give you a combination of herbal tinctures to take several times a day, and perhaps recommend that you delay trying to conceive for three months while your body is strengthened.

Chinese Herbs

Western medical herbalism differs from Chinese herbal medicine in the nature of the plants involved, which may be grown in China and are often used in conjunction with acupuncture. Zita West, a former midwife with the U.K.'s National Health Service and an acupuncturist, uses a combination of Chinese herbs, nutritional therapy, and acupuncture, and she reports great success in treating hormonal disturbances, including PCOS: "The whole principle of Chinese medicine is that you need to be at maximum strength to conceive," says West. There's actually more research evidence available regarding these plants than there is for Western medical herbalism.[f]

Chinese herbs can help improve general health and readiness for conception, and they can be generally supportive during infertility treatment. For example, a study at the Department of Gynecology, Second Affiliated Hospital, Hebei Medical College, Shijiazhuang, reported the treatment of 149 cases with menstrual disorders.[147] The results showed that ovulation rates were significantly higher in the group treated with traditional Chinese herbs and clomiphene (see the Glossary) than that of the group who were treated with just one or the other, showing that a combination of Western and Chinese herbal medicine may have advantages.

Herbal Treatments

The following treatments have all been used with varying degrees of success by women with PCOS who have fertility problems or irregular periods, and you may find that these plants will be recommended if you visit a herbalist for a custom prescription.

Remember that these are powerful substances, and large amounts of any herb or dietary supplement should only be taken under the supervision of a doctor, qualified consultant, or herbalist, preferably one experienced in treating women with PCOS.

1. **Agnus castus** (vitex/chasteberry tree) has been shown to stimulate and normalize the function of the pituitary gland, which helps balance hormone output from the ovaries and stimulate ovulation.[148] Agnus castus also keeps prolactin secretion in check for rats, which is helpful since excessive prolactin can prevent ovulation. Also called *vitex,* this plant is used as an herbal treatment for infertility, particularly in cases with established luteal phase defect (shortened second half of the menstrual cycle) and high levels of prolactin. In one trial, 48 women, ages 23–39, who were diagnosed with infertility took vitex once a day for three months[149-51]—of the 48 women, 7 became pregnant during the trial, and 25 experienced normalized progesterone levels, which may increase the chances for pregnancy.

In another double-blind trial, significantly more infertile women became pregnant after taking a product with vitex as the main ingredient (the other ingredients were homeopathic preparations), than did those who took a placebo.[152] The amount used in this trial was 30 drops of fluid extract twice a day, for a total of 1.8 ml per day. This specific preparation isn't available in the United States, but there are many tinctures of vitex available in health-food stores or from medical herbalists.

Some doctors recommend taking 40 drops of a liquid extract of vitex each morning with water, and approximately 35–40 mg of encapsulated powdered vitex (one capsule taken in the morning) provides a similar amount of the herb. Vitex should be discontinued once a woman becomes pregnant.

2. **Black cohosh** has a balancing effect on hormones and is often prescribed by medical herbalists for women with PCOS and irregular cycles.[153]

3. **Dong quai,** a Chinese herb also called *angelica*, is well known as a tonic for the female reproductive system because it regulates hormonal control and improves the rhythm of the menstrual cycle.[154]

4. **False unicorn root** (chamaelirium luteum) also acts as a tonic for the reproductive system, but it can also help regulate periods. It's often found in women's herbal compounds because of its balancing effect on hormones.

5. A Japanese study has found that the **licorice** plant helped women with PCOS and irregular periods. However, only use it under professional supervision because it can only be taken to help regulate your cycle—not when you're trying to get pregnant.

6. **Red-raspberry leaf** is a native European shrub that's been used by women for centuries as an herbal tonic, usually in the form of tea. Chemical analysis reports that the herb contains estrogenlike compounds that can promote menstrual regularity and fertility.

7. The herbal medicine **sairei-to** may be a useful treatment for women with PCOS and irregular cycles, according to research at the department of obstetrics and gynecology at Nippon Kokan Hospital in Kagawa, Japan.[155]

8. A study in the *International Journal of Fertility* showed encouraging results when infertile women were treated with **shakuyaku-kanzo-to (TJ-68).**[156]

9. **Shatawari** is popular Ayurvedic tonic used by some women to help normalize the hormonal imbalances of PCOS that cause irregular cycles.

10. **Siberian ginseng** is believed to help your body adapt to stress and balance blood sugar, and it's often recommended to women with PCOS and irregular cycles. It isn't recommended,

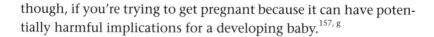

though, if you're trying to get pregnant because it can have potentially harmful implications for a developing baby.[157, 8]

11. **Unicorn root** ("true"—as opposed to "false"—unicorn root) is a North American herb said to be useful for women with delayed or absent periods. **White Peony** is another herb, like unicorn root, that may help normalize the balance or hormones.

12. When women with irregular periods were treated with the Japanese herb **unkei-to** in a controlled study, the rate of menstrual improvement for women with PCOS was 50 percent.[158]

13. **Wild Yam** is an anti-inflammatory agent with a weak hormonal activity in the body, which can improve menstrual function and fertility.

In addition to the benefits of these remedies, herbs can also be a powerful force in balancing insulin levels and reducing insulin resistance in PCOS, according to Dr. Ann Walker, medical herbalist and senior lecturer in human nutrition at the University of Reading. When treating many women with PCOS, as well as diabetic patients in conjunction with the local hospitals, Dr. Walker often uses **bilberry, goat's rue, cinnamon,** and **fenugreek** for people with insulin problems, as well as **holy basil** for more extreme cases.

Reflexology

Many women with PCOS have found reflexology helpful, saying that it relaxes them and helps their cycles become more regular. This treatment feels like a vigorous foot massage, during which the therapist stimulates specific points on your foot that are thought to link into energy channels called *meridians* running throughout your body (a tenet of Chinese medicine and acupuncture). Pressing one point in the foot influences the energy flow around all the other organs and body areas that run along that meridian.

"Reflexology is one of the most effective ways of rebalancing the entire endocrine system," says U.K.-based practitioner Jacqui Garnier (see the Resource Guide), who has PCOS herself and uses reflexology to help other women. "It is particularly successful when used in conjunction with a healthy diet and lifestyle. As a balancing treatment, it has been known to have success rates as high as 88 percent in infertility; it can regulate cycles, tone the uterus, encourage ovulation, and improve the function of the ovaries; it can balance heavy and painful periods and reduce the stress so often associated with coping with the symptoms of PCOS."

There's been little research done on the efficacy of reflexology in infertility, although a small trial in Denmark examined 108 women with an average age of 30 who had been trying to conceive for an average of 6.7 years. Many dropped out of the trial, but 19 of the remaining 61 conceived within six months of completing the treatment.

Aromatherapy

While there's little evidence to suggest that aromatherapy can directly combat infertility, it can certainly help alleviate the emotional stresses associated with infertility and going through fertility treatment.

Work carried out by Dr. Gary Schwartz, former professor of psychology and psychiatry at Yale University, found that, by themselves, the aromas of some essential oils affect the nervous system and even reduce blood pressure. (The scent of spice apple, for example, was found to reduce blood pressure by an average of three to five points in healthy volunteers.)

Infertility problems can create enormous emotional stresses, and certainly aromatherapy is an excellent way to help counter such stress and induce relaxation. And, as we've seen, stress does affect your hormones and insulin balance—extreme stress can delay or even stop your periods. So although there's no clinical evidence yet, it seems that the stress-relieving effects of aromatherapy are not to be dismissed.

U.K. aromatherapist and reflexologist Frances Box specializes in fertility treatments and believes that aromatherapy oils do, in and of themselves, have something to offer in increasing fertility. After all, they're potent plant oils that get into the bloodstream through the skin (much like the medication in nicotine patches), and they can have a chemical effect on the body.

"Rose is known as the queen of oils. It's traditionally used for infertility because it contains a substance similar to estrogen," she says, also noting that "relaxation is a large part of the process." Box uses oils such as lavender, ylang ylang, clary sage, and marjoram, which work to relax the nervous system. Many of her clients have had or are having IVF, and ideally, she likes to carry out her therapies alongside it.

She explains, "IVF is very stressful, what with counting days, taking temperatures and samples, and being on [pins and needles] about the outcome. So my first role is to relax clients who are usually depressed, anxious, and stressed to the hilt. When you're stressed, it doesn't just affect your mind, but your hormones too. Prolactin, for example, is a hormone which is influenced by stress, which can affect a woman's fertility. I believe that if you reduce stress, you improve your chances of fertility."

A therapeutic massage combined with carefully selected essential oils certainly makes aromatherapy an excellent aid in countering the effects of stress and inducing relaxation. Massage improves the blood circulation in several ways without putting additional strain on the heart: It helps the flow of blood through the veins, stimulates the nerves that control the blood vessels, and relaxes tense muscles and tight connective tissues that may have been constricting the circulatory system, thus enabling better blood flow.

It's for this reason that soothing massage reduces emotional tension, induces relaxation, and calms stress-related conditions, leading to improvements in your general health and well-being.

Acupuncture

Perhaps one of the best-researched complementary therapies, acupuncture has been found by many women with PCOS to be most helpful for kick-starting absent periods and regulating cycles. Some research has also shown that it can have a balancing effect on hormones, which is particularly good for women with PCOS.[159–160] Studies on the benefits of Chinese medicine in general for women with irregular periods have also produced encouraging results.[161] Traditional acupuncturists treat the whole person rather than a disease, and attempt to get to the root cause of the problem instead of just treating the symptoms. As with other holistic practitioners, they'll also consider all lifestyle and environmental factors before beginning.

"Acupuncture is based on the principle of influencing the flow of vital energy around the body using needles. It is deceptively simple, correcting imbalances to assist the body's own recuperative powers to restore harmony and vital function," explains Susan Birch, who's been an acupuncturist for 12 years, specializing in fertility for the last 4. She recently opened The Center for Optimum Fertility in France, where couples can go for a four-day residential stay in the French countryside. The center aims to offer an environment of deep relaxation as clients undergo treatment.

"Acupuncture boosts fertility as it helps to invigorate the flow of blood and energy to the lower abdominal area. For women, it will assist in regulating the menstrual cycle, boost ovulation, and improve fertility. I have had great success in treating endometriosis, blocked fallopian tubes, ovarian cysts, and infertility-related hormonal imbalances, like PCOS," she says.

There's published evidence to show that acupuncture works for problems such as back pain, toothaches, and migraines, and a clinical trial published in *Gynecological Endocrinology* in 1992 suggests that acupuncture can help with infertility.[162] Following a complete gynecologic endocrinologic examination, 45 infertile women suffering from menstrual irregularity and infertility were treated with auricular acupuncture (treatment of points on the ear). Results were compared to those of 45 women who received hormone treatment. Both groups were matched for age, duration of infertility, body mass index, previous pregnancies, menstrual cycle, and the presence of any blockages in the fallopian tubes.

Women treated with acupuncture had 22 pregnancies, whereas women treated with hormones had 20 pregnancies. It was also noted that side effects were observed only during hormone treatment, and various disorders of the autonomic nervous system normalized during acupuncture. The study concluded that "auricular acupuncture seems to offer a valuable alternative therapy for female infertility due to hormone disorders," being more effective than hormone therapy and with no side effects.

> "My endocrinologist sent me for an ultrasound and diagnosed PCOS from the results. I was devastated because he implied that I would most likely need fertility treatment to get pregnant. He offered me metformin, but I declined. Instead, I began a strict healthy-eating program, went to the gym four times a week, and took a number of supplements, including vitex. I had weekly acupuncture as well. By accident, my close friend mentioned my diagnosis to her acupuncturist, who also suffers from PCOS, and she that said she could help me. After three weeks on the diet and just three acupuncture sessions, I could feel a huge difference. My skin cleared up, I had more energy, and I lost around ten pounds— I felt amazing. Two weeks later, I ovulated, and I expected my period to come around a couple weeks after that, so it was a great and very happy surprise when I did a home pregnancy test and found out that I was going to have a baby." — Eve

Hypnotherapy: The Mind/Body Connection

Hypnotherapy works on the premise that there are two states of consciousness—the conscious and the subconscious—that may be working against each other. "I believe that while a woman might consciously want a baby, her subconscious may be stopping her from getting pregnant," says Elizabeth Muir, a clinical psychologist based in London who specializes in helping women who have "unexplained infertility." "Most of the women I see have psychosomatic infertility related to conflicts, or unresolved issues about having a baby. A combination of counseling and hypnotherapy can remove these problems," she says. Muir also believes that if women have psychological blocks about having a baby, their bodies will manifest this resistance in conditions such as endometriosis or polycystic ovaries. Muir's clients range from ages 37 to 45, and she claims a 45 percent success rate, based on live births that resulted from conceptions taking place within her ten suggested sessions of treatment, or within one year after completion of treatment.

There's huge pressure on women these days to have the perfect life, body, job, partner, and family, but you may have doubts and insecurities about motherhood and feel pressured to conceive by those around you. It's important to find out what you really want. "Subconscious worries can prevent conception, so hypnotherapy can deal with doubts about your future role as a mother," confirms Julie Gerland, a clinical hypnotherapist and founder of the Center of Universal Unity in Hong Kong. She also specializes in emotional clearing, which she believes is necessary for parenting.

There was some evidence published in the *European Journal of Clinical Hypnosis* in 1994 that hypnotherapy could help in medically unexplained, functional, and psychosomatic infertility. If you're interested in this option, you may also want to try a hypnotherapy CD called "Prepare to Conceive," which has been developed by Nourish, a natural-fertility program that encourages couples to improve their emotional and physical health before planning for a baby (also see the Resource Guide).

Homeopathy

"Homeopathy is a method of helping the body heal itself using very diluted substances—many derived from plants, which at higher doses would produce the symptoms being treated—we explain it by saying 'like treats like,'" says Annetta Kershaw, a qualified homeopath practicing in Keighley in Yorkshire, U.K. If you remember that vaccination works on the same principle, it can help explain the logic behind this system of medicine, although scientists are puzzled about how it actually produces some very effective results.

Although Kershaw has great success in helping women conceive, she does not claim to "specialize" in PCOS-related infertility because by its very nature, homeopathy treats the whole person rather than the symptom. "We would see infertility as simply a symptom, and we would concentrate on looking at the imbalances of the whole person—emotional, physical, and mental—which could be causing the infertility. Therefore, there is no simple recipe to treat infertility because every individual is unique," she says.

This is why homeopaths will take a detailed life and case history from every patient, and why a range of "constitutional" remedies exist, which correspond to different types of people. If a homeopath can find your constitutional remedy by working out what type of person you are (emotionally, physically, and in the way you relate to the world around you), this is thought to help unlock some of your basic underlying health problems. In addition, there are many homoeopathic remedies designed to relieve specific symptoms— anything from nausea to acne.

Homeopathic remedies help your system clear itself of any imbalances and are used to treat symptoms such as irregular menstrual cycles. Some will target the uterus or ovaries, and others will treat any mental or emotional disparities that your therapist may think are keeping you from conceiving.

In a 2000 German study, 30 infertile women with hormonal problems were given homeopathic remedies, while a matched group was treated with placebo.[163] The results for the homeopathic group were encouraging, and increasingly, medical experts are suggesting homeopathy as a complement or alternative to conventional medicine.[164]

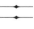

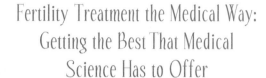

Chapter Five

Fertility Treatment the Medical Way:
Getting the Best That Medical
Science Has to Offer

Hopefully, by the time you read this chapter, you'll have a better understanding of how the complex and delicate balance of your hormones can be upset by your diet and lifestyle. However, when you're trying to get pregnant and nothing seems to be happening, it's easy to panic. So in this chapter, we'll tell you where and how to get conventional help for fertility problems, as well as the kinds of treatments most likely to be recommended if you have PCOS.

Being in a healthy state of mind and body will increase your chances of success with any fertility therapy. You're most likely to get pregnant when your body is at maximum harmony—that is, in hormonal balance. Follow the advice in our preconception plan, take care of yourself, live well, and above all, be happy.

The Cost of Infertility

The first step to successfully managing your fertility treatment is to find a good doctor. You need to find a fertility specialist: someone who treats women and couples with fertility problems and who, ideally, has experience treating women with PCOS. This choice may be greatly influenced by financial factors.

> *"Having a baby is the most important thing in my life right now. It's already cost us more than we can afford, but however much it ends up being, I'm going to make it happen."* — Toni, 39 years old

> *"When I saw the cost of treatment, I was shocked. I'm a nurse, and my partner is unemployed—we can't get our hands on money like that. Right now, I just don't know what I'm going to do. I do sometimes wonder, though, if this just isn't meant to be."* — Elizabeth, 26 years old

Infertility is now big business in both the U.K. and the U.S., and about 85 percent of fertility treatments are carried out by private clinics. If you have PCOS and want to have a baby, you may feel very vulnerable and could end up spending a great deal of money to find out why you're having difficulties, and then spend much more on treatment. The average cost of a single IVF (in vitro fertilization) treatment in the United States is close to $5,000.

Long waiting lists aren't good news if you have PCOS and time isn't on your side. So what can you do if waiting and remortgaging your home aren't options? Fortunately, many women with PCOS won't actually need the more advanced and expensive treatments such as IVF. Preliminary testing and ovulation-boosting drugs (such as Clomid) may be all that's needed, and most of these simpler procedures can be provided and prescribed at a private fertility clinic. If this is the case, it will be more affordable, costing hundreds, rather than thousands, of dollars.

Finding a Fertility Specialist

Unfortunately, some fertility clinics are more ethical and honest with their clients than others, so it's worth taking the time to choose one you feel comfortable with. If you decide to pay for independent care rather than using your health insurance or HMO (in the United States) or going to a state-run clinic (in the U.K.), you'll have more control and the opportunity to select an environment you feel happy in. Some medical practices are small and friendly and allow you to see the same doctor each time, whereas others are big, hospital-based units.

When choosing a private clinic (assuming that you decide to do so), try to find out about their success rates: Shop around, call and ask for several brochures, and contact an infertility organization, such as RESOLVE for advice about choosing a clinic. In the U.S., the American Society of Reproductive Medicine is a nonprofit trade organization that offers information on finding a doctor. You also could ask your family health-care provider to recommend a clinic or ask other women with PCOS via support groups. Choose three or four places that appeal to you and aren't too far away, and then visit them or ask to speak to a senior consultant or counselor on the phone.

Questions to Ask When Deciding on a Clinic

- Are the consultants fully qualified?

- Will your specialist be an ob-gyn who has additional training in reproductive endocrinology?

- Do the consultants have experience treating women with PCOS?

- What treatments and tests do they offer?

- Do they have any age restrictions?

- Do they have a waiting list?

- How successful are they in treating women with PCOS?

- Do they offer 24-hour service so that you can be seen right away for emergencies if necessary?

- Will you be closely monitored while taking fertility drugs?

- What are their success rates in live (sometimes called *take home*) births?

- What are the costs?

- What might be covered by insurance?

- Are there any hidden fees?

Try to meet the specialist who'll be in charge of your treatment before you make your final choice, and then ask *yourself* some questions: Do I feel comfortable with them? Do they inspire me with confidence? What does my partner think?

Although clinics are supposed to report accurate success rates, this may not always be the case, especially in the United States, where the industry generates $2 billion a year. If you're thinking of registering somewhere, never sign up immediately. Take your time and do your research: Speak to former patients; find out about the doctors treating you; contact advisory boards; and seek second, third, and fourth opinions. This is a huge decision, and it's vital that you feel comfortable with it.

How to Get the Most from Your Doctor

If your doctor recommends taking fertility drugs when there's a full waiting room and he or she clearly doesn't have the time to discuss PCOS at length, you may feel pressured to make major decisions after only a quick conversation. If that's the case, don't be intimidated. Prepare for your appointments ahead of time by writing down what you need to ask. When you're at the office, take notes and maybe even bring along a friend (who can prompt you if you forget anything). If you feel that you'll need more time, don't be afraid to ask the receptionist for a double appointment or to schedule you during your doctor's quietest time.

If you're concerned about the advice you've been given, there's nothing wrong with asking for a second opinion. Remember, it's your doctor's responsibility to provide all the information you need, and you should never feel obligated to make a decision on the spot. Instead, go home and get in touch with your PCOS support group to help find more information.

If the worst happens, and your doctor is dismissive or rude about your concerns, try to remain calm and assertive. Patients who assert themselves get better care, so be reasonable but firm. If you just don't get along with your health-care provider or fertility specialist, you can stay registered with the same organization, but ask to see someone else when you call for an appointment—or you can change clinics altogether.

If you aren't happy with the care you receive, tell someone, such as another doctor, about the cause of your concern. Alternatively, ask about the procedures for complaints. In the United States, you may also contact your state medical board for help.

The way to secure the best care for yourself is to take control. Learn to stand up for yourself in consultations and give yourself all the time and space you need to make one of the most important decisions of your life.

Methods for Monitoring Ovulation

To achieve pregnancy, you need to know if and when you're ovulating, and the most reliable way to determine this is by undergoing a series of diagnostic tests. These are usually done in conjunction with examination of your cervical mucus or when taking your temperature (see page 29 in Chapter 2).

Transvaginal ultrasound is an important tool for diagnosing PCOS and determining whether you're ovulating. In this procedure, the doctor inserts a handheld cylindrical instrument called a *transducer* into your vagina. It uses sound waves to produce images so that your ovaries and uterine lining can be measured. In this way, the doctor can see exactly how many follicles are developing and how big they are. To be considered the optimal size for conception, they should measure about 16–22 mm in diameter, and in order to sustain a pregnancy, the uterine lining should be about 10–12 mm thick.

If you aren't having periods, you may be given some progesterone or progestins to induce one, and 21 days later (or, if your periods are regular, 7 days after you think you may have ovulated), you may also be given a progesterone test. This will tell you if an egg was released from the ovary. If it was, your progesterone level should be significantly higher, but if levels are low, it's likely that the egg wasn't released.

Some doctors suggest that you have an ultrasound, a progesterone test, *and* a postcoital test, which is a bit like having a pap smear a few hours after sex in order to see if your partner's sperm is surviving in your cervical mucus. If you did ovulate successfully, your period will begin 14 days after ovulation, and if it doesn't . . . you could already be pregnant!

If you didn't ovulate, however, your doctor may suggest that you try another progestin cycle, or he or she may suggest fertility medication to induce ovulation.

Fertility Treatments to Induce
Ovulation in Women with PCOS

Most of the drugs used to induce ovulation have unpleasant side effects ranging from nausea to mood swings to insomnia, so make sure to ask your specialist to keep you fully informed. Also, bear in mind that some studies indicate that fertility medication to induce ovulation may be associated with ovarian cancer and ovarian hyperstimulation syndrome—a rare-but-serious condition in which the ovaries enlarge as a result of fertility treatment and can cause damage not just to future fertility, but to other organs as well.[165]

"It's common to have an exaggerated response to ovarian stimulation with PCOS," says syndrome expert Dr. Sam Thatcher. "So if you've got PCOS, you need to be aware that your chances of ovarian hyperstimulation may increase because there are already lots of partially developed follicles on your ovary, all in suspended animation, and fertility drugs are more likely to stimulate multiple follicles."

Proceed with Caution

There are still glaring gaps in our knowledge about what dangers fertility drugs may pose and whether the benefits outweigh the risks. Clinical trials haven't been done to establish links between several rounds of commonly prescribed fertility drugs (such as Clomid) and ovarian cancer, but many experts believe that such a connection exists.

In 2003, the journal *Fertility and Sterility* published a National Institutes of Health study showing that women who'd taken Pergonal-type drugs had a risk of breast cancer that was two to three times greater than those who hadn't. Cancer, however is not the only threat hanging over those who take fertility drugs; they also carry the risk of anxiety, depression, and chronic physical distress, such as chest pain, hives, and other severe, unexplained pain.

Many questions remain unanswered about the uses and side effects of fertility drugs. Perhaps this information will be discovered one day, but for now, bear in mind that their use is still experimental, and you should proceed with extreme caution. For all the hope that reproductive medicine can bring, it also breaks many hearts and carries risks that are as yet unknown.

Using Fertility Drugs

The major benefit of taking fertility medication is that you have a better chance of ovulating and getting pregnant when you do. These drugs work by stimulating egg production, encouraging ovulation, or by stabilizing hormone levels that could be inhibiting ovulation. A number of women with PCOS find that ovulation-inducing drugs work, but not all medications are successful for everyone.

"We'd been trying to get pregnant for four years, and once my 30th birthday was approaching, I decided it was time to see a doctor. All I'd ever wanted was to be a mother, and even as a little girl, I used to rock my little sister and sing her to sleep. I was the most sought-after babysitter with my friends, but now I wanted to have a baby myself. I was diagnosed with PCOS and put on a course of Clomid therapy with a series of ultrasounds to determine the growth and size of my follicle. When it was large enough (a whopping 24mm!), the doctor injected me in my hip, explaining that I needed this to help the egg release from its follicle. That shot really hurt, and for a few days afterward, I was sore. I expected the treatment to take a while and wasn't looking forward to another injection, so you can imagine our shock when the pregnancy test was positive." — Elizabeth, 32 years old

"I'd heard so much about how wonderful Clomid can be for women with PCOS, and my sister, who's also got PCOS, got pregnant on her second cycle of the drug, so I started my fertility treatment with high hopes. But when the fourth cycle failed, I realized

that Clomid wasn't going to be a miracle worker for me. My doctor suggested a final course of it, but this time with metformin, too. It worked: I'm the proud mother of a baby boy, age three. Four months ago, I had another course of Clomid with metformin and found out that I'm pregnant again—with twins. I couldn't be happier!" — Sonia, 36 years old

You can maximize your chance of success with medical treatments by also using complementary therapies that can help encourage regular ovulation, such as acupuncture, reflexology, herbalism, hypnotherapy, and relaxation techniques.[166] Do make sure, though, that you work with a qualified practitioner and that you tell your fertility specialist what you're doing in case there are any contraindications.

Clomiphene Citrate
(brand names Clomid and Serophene)

"Clomid is usually the first-line therapy for induction of ovulation in PCOS," says Dr. Thatcher. The drug works by causing the body to produce more follicle-stimulating hormone (FSH) and luteinizing hormone (LH) to promote egg growth. Once the brain senses increased estrogen levels, it signals the LH surge that results in ovulation.

It can take a few cycles to determine the right dosage for you, but Clomid shouldn't be taken for more than six months at a time. There are several potential side effects, including headaches, depression, fatigue, and a 5 to 10 percent risk of twins or triplets (Clomid increases the number of preovulatory follicles and ovulations and therefore the chance of multiple pregnancy).

More serious side effects include ovarian enlargement or hyperstimulation. If there are any changes in your vision, or if you suffer from severe headaches when taking this medication, tell your doctor immediately. It can also have a negative impact on fertility by causing your cervical mucus to become hostile to sperm.

Because of the potential side effects, use the lowest amount that results in ovulation. It's standard to begin with 50 mg (one tablet). Success is usually achieved by taking at least 150 mg (three tablets a day), but the "more is better" rule doesn't apply, since higher doses can actually *prevent* pregnancy rather than *promote* it. The dose needs to be adjusted according to body weight, with heavier patients needing higher levels. Clomid may be started on day two, three, four, or five of your cycle and is usually given over five days. A recent conference in San Diego looked at different ways to give this drug to women with PCOS but concluded that there's no one regimen that's better than another.

If you haven't gotten pregnant after five or six cycles of treatment, this therapy clearly isn't working. Research suggests that about two thirds of women taking Clomid ovulate within four cycles, and some studies show that about 35 percent achieve pregnancy.[167] If your doctor doesn't recommend a change at this point, it might be wise to seek another opinion. Although this medication is fairly inexpensive, costing around $120 per treatment cycle, studies show that there's an increased risk of ovarian cancer after 12 or more cycles, and women with PCOS must be followed with particular care.[168]

Most doctors are unwilling to prescribe more than six cycles at any one time, but every case needs to be discussed with your health-care provider or a fertility specialist to ensure that the right decision is made.

Unfortunately, many women with PCOS are Clomid-resistant and don't ovulate even when taking the maximum dose. But there are new ways to look at monitoring its effectiveness, so talk to your specialist about these options before you begin. Recent studies have also shown that when taken with an insulin sensitizer (such as metformin), Clomid significantly increases the chances of ovulation and pregnancy.[169] Other studies suggest that using estrogen supplementation with Clomid increased pregnancy rates, perhaps by encouraging growth of the lining of the womb and increasing the implantation rate—although some doctors don't think that estrogen supplementation is helpful.[170]

A word on safety for the baby: Nearly 50 years of experience with this drug has shown that the rate of birth defects with its use isn't any higher than that of the general population.

Gonadotropins

Gonadotropins are drugs that stimulate your ovaries to release eggs by supplying your body with an extra amount of FSH or LH (the hormones that start egg production). Possible side effects include bloating, nausea, depression, and hot flashes. There's also an increased risk of ovarian hyperstimulation (around 1 percent) and multiple pregnancy (around 20 percent). The most common gonadotropins are FSH, human menopausal gonadotropin (HMG), and human chorionic gonadotropin (HCG).

1. **FSH (follicle-stimulating hormone)** controls ovulation in partnership with LH. Because women with PCOS often have an elevated LH level, sometimes pure FSH is given to balance the ratio. Once there are adequate levels of estrogen and the follicle develops, an HCG shot is given to release the egg. There are different types of FSH available, but those most often prescribed are Fertinex, Gonal-F, and Follistim. FSH is given by daily injection and is usually expensive. Side effects can include mood swings and ovarian hyperstimulation.

2. More commonly known as Pergonal and Repronex, **Human Menopausal Gonadotropin (HMG)** medication is an extract from the urine of menopausal women and contains LH and FSH, which stimulate ovulation. It's given by injection, usually in the thigh or buttocks. Some research suggests that about 90 percent of women ovulate using HMG, but only 60 percent conceive. Side effects can include mood swings, and if not monitored properly, there's an increased risk of ovarian hyperstimulation, along with multiple pregnancy.

3. **Human Chorionic Gonadotropin (HCG)** is the hormone that makes an ovary release its dominant follicle (the ripest one), and also helps keep your womb lining in place if you get pregnant. The drug HCG is used with other fertility medications including Clomid, FSH, and HMG to promote ovulation by triggering the LH surge. There's an increased risk of ovarian hyperstimulation and cyst formation, and in some women with PCOS, a follicle develops well with other fertility medications, but the egg is never released. If this happens to you (the follicle appears ripe but LH fails to trigger release), your doctor can give you an injection of HCG to cause ovulation.

Insulin Sensitizers

Insulin sensitizers such as Avandia and metformin are considered one of the most effective methods for treating infertility in women with PCOS, since they can bring insulin levels into balance. "Treatment with insulin-sensitizing drugs (metformin) has shown promising results in preliminary studies, including reinstated menstrual periods and improved fertility," says PCOS expert Gabor Kovacs.[171–2]

Many women who couldn't ovulate on other fertility medications achieve success using insulin sensitizers because they decrease insulin resistance, which has a positive effect on ovarian function. As mentioned earlier, studies show that by using these drugs in combination with Clomid or another fertility medication, over half of women with PCOS will ovulate.

Your doctor may only prescribe them if you have insulin resistance, but many women with PCOS have found the medication helpful even if they only have borderline or normal glucose levels and aren't insulin resistant. Talk to your doctor to find out if this option makes sense for you.

If you're wondering whether it's safe to take metformin when you're trying to get pregnant, it's worth remembering that with insulin-altering drugs such as metformin, the potential benefits can exceed the risks.[173] We've seen how metformin can increase the chances of pregnancy in women with PCOS who are insulin resistant, and research also suggests that its use by diabetic women throughout their pregnancies showed no measurable increase in miscarriage and birth defects.[174–5, h]

However, these drugs aren't entirely risk free (side effects include gastrointestinal symptoms, diarrhea, nausea, bloating, and loss of appetite), but then neither is PCOS in pregnancy, or gestational diabetes, which is more likely in women with PCOS. (For information on gestational diabetes, see Chapter 6.)

Ovarian Surgery

This is only an option if other medications have failed. There are two types of ovarian surgery: ovarian drilling (also known as *diathermy*), and wedge resection. Surgery can't cure PCOS, but it can promote ovulation to increase your chances of pregnancy.

Ovarian drilling is an outpatient laparoscopic procedure in which a laser is used to pierce the thickened coat of the ovary. The surgeon then uses the laser to penetrate the cysts on each ovary; after which, fluid is drained, eliminating many of the cysts. In turn, testosterone production is lowered, causing a decrease in LH.

About 80 percent of women undergoing the procedure will ovulate, and about 30 to 40 percent will get pregnant. Being close to your ideal weight will improve your chances of success. Possible risks include the normal complications of surgery, along with possible adhesions and destruction of the ovary.

However, don't worry if you've had diathermy and it hasn't been successful. If the procedure didn't result in complications and you had a good recovery, there's still the option of fertility drug treatment afterward.

Wedge resection is a major procedure that's rarely performed today. It involves the surgical removal of cysts and can increase the chances of ovulation, but it carries with it a high risk of adhesions that can prevent pregnancy.

Assisted Reproductive Technologies

"When every other option failed, my doctor suggested IVF. I had no idea what to expect, and in retrospect, it's probably a good thing I didn't. First, there were the injectable drugs to stimulate my ovary, which hurt and made me feel sick. I had countless scans and blood tests to determine if my eggs were big enough and to see if my hormone levels were right. Then there was one last injection to help me ovulate. Exactly 36 hours later, I had what's known as a follicle aspiration, where a needle is passed through the vaginal wall and an egg is removed from the follicles by suction, assisted by the use of ultrasound fluid. Immediately after aspiration, the egg is isolated from the follicular fluid and placed with my husband's sperm into an incubator in a culture dish. I'm a bit of a coward when it comes to needles and things, so I opted for general anesthetic because I've heard that all this can be really painful.

"About 48 hours later, the egg and sperm had formed an embryo, which was placed in my womb. I wanted general anesthesia again for implantation, but my doctor reassured me that it wasn't necessary, and he was right—I didn't feel a thing. Then came the hardest part of all: the waiting. For two weeks, I was a prisoner in my own home. My doctor had told me to carry on with my life as usual, but I couldn't. I didn't want to do anything that might harm my baby. When the phone call came saying that it hadn't worked, my world collapsed, but I immediately signed up for a second round of treatment. That didn't work either. On my third round, I began to wonder if this was ever going to work, and my husband and I started to consider adoption. After that third implantation, I went about my normal routine, convinced that I wasn't pregnant. Then the phone rang. I went into shock: We'd done it—I was pregnant." — Jane, 37 years old

Some women with PCOS who aren't successful at getting pregnant using the treatments already described turn to assisted reproductive technology (ART). These procedures can be extremely expensive and carry with them the risks of multiple births, ovarian hyperstimulation, and high rates of miscarriage.[176] As always with fertility treatments, the best advice is to proceed with extreme caution. Success rates are variable and depend on many factors, including your age, your partner's sperm quality and quantity, how experienced your doctor is, the quality of your eggs, and the number of cycles attempted.

Although many pregnancies with techniques such as IVF and gamete-fallopian transfer (GIFT) do occur on the first cycle, chances of success appear to be equal each time through the first four tries, and the average couple will undergo two or three attempts before a successful pregnancy. Although there are always exceptions, the pregnancy rate starts to decline after the fourth cycle, and it's reasonable to review your options with your doctor at that time and think about stopping the process.

Research has suggested that women with PCOS tend to produce many eggs, but still have lower fetilization rates with ART. "Certainly, we know that eggs from women with PCOS are not always 'good,'" says PCOS expert Dr. Samuel Thatcher. "There is evidence to suggest that eggs extracted from the small cysts of PCOS ovaries have much less capacity to undergo development than do eggs from follicles of similar size in women without PCOS."[177] So if you're thinking about ART, you should consult your doctor or fertility specialist for an evaluation to assess your chances of succeeding. Here are some of the techniques that might be discussed:

1. In **IVF (in vitro fertilization)**, the woman's eggs are fertilized with her partner's sperm in a lab, and the resulting very young embryos are placed back into the womb so that they can implant in the lining there. Sometimes, if several attempts have been made, IVF is combined with "assisted hatching," in which a needle or chemical is used to make a tiny hole in the embryo's casing so that it can attach itself more easily to the uterine lining. The transfer takes only a few minutes and involves placing a small plastic tube through the cervix into the uterine cavity. No anesthesia is required, and there's usually minimal, if any, discomfort.

2. Although very popular in the '80s and '90s, **GIFT (gamete-fallopian transfer)** is now used much less frequently than IVF. In this procedure, eggs are taken from the ovary, then sperm and eggs are simultaneously placed into the fallopian tubes (the structures through which the eggs travel from the ovary to the uterus).

3. **ZIFT (zygote interfallopian transfer)** involves removing eggs from the ovary and then fertilizing them with sperm in the lab. A day later, the embryos are placed into the fallopian tube.

4. In **IUI (intrauterine insemination)**, egg production is stimulated through the use of fertility medications and monitored closely by the doctor. When ovulation occurs, sperm is deposited directly into the uterus to shorten the distance to the ovary.

5. A single sperm is injected into an egg through a very tiny needle for **Intracytoplasmic Sperm Injection.** Two days later, the resulting embryo is transferred into the uterus.

6. In a different approach, the mother-to-be can receive **donor eggs**—that is, eggs from another woman. They're fertilized in the lab with the sperm from a partner or donor and then placed into the uterus. Although the woman receiving them isn't the genetic mother, she will be the birth mother.

Helping Yourself

Adam Balen, consultant gynecologist and obstetrician and specialist in reproductive medicine and surgery at Leeds General Infirmary, U.K., is a great believer in individualism when it comes to fertility treatment for PCOS. "Some treatments, like Clomid, help women with PCOS get pregnant; but PCOS is a complex disorder, and there isn't one fertility treatment or approach per se. You have to treat each patient with PCOS as a unique individual to find what works best for her. Much will depend on body weight," he says.

"These days we should start with metformin and then add in fertility drugs, like Clomid, if ovulation isn't happening."

PCOS is complex, and finding the right treatment for you will take time and patience, but one thing remains certain: Whatever the treatment, you can help yourself. As we've seen, research has shown that even a basic multivitamin and mineral during fertility treatment can improve your chances of success with IVF. The complex procedures can leave you feeling quite powerless, but healthful diet and lifestyle changes such those recommended in Chapters 2 and 3 can enhance the power of any process, boost your energy, and, best of all, give you a feeling of control.

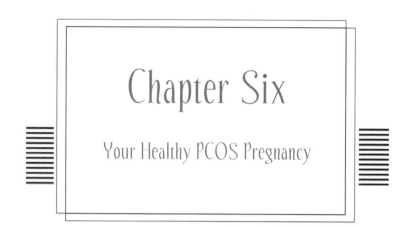

Chapter Six

Your Healthy PCOS Pregnancy

The great majority of women with PCOS can, and do, get pregnant. When the blessed event finally happens, it can bring a whole bunch of emotions to the surface, from excitement to disbelief to panic to joy. And then, as you get used to the idea that you're going to be parents, you start wanting to read books about staying healthy throughout your pregnancy. After all, you've heard of those extra risks of miscarriage and getting diabetes because of your PCOS. You may worry that if you put on excess pounds, you'll never be able to lose it because of the weight trap of this condition. And is the diet you've been following in order to keep your hormones in balance the best diet to continue with now that you're having a baby?

But wait a minute—a lot of pregnancy books don't mention PCOS, so how do you know which parts of them are relevant to you?

We hope that this chapter brings you the PCOS-focused information you need to add to the general facts already out there in other books and Websites. The basic ideas are the same—healthy eating, gentle exercise, and taking care of yourself—but there are some extra steps you can follow with PCOS to ensure that you and your baby are the healthiest you can be.

> "I first suspected something was up when I stopped taking the Pill last summer. I'd never really suffered from acne before, nor had my periods ever really been too irregular. They were never exactly like clockwork, but when I came off the Pill, I'd skip one month and then get it between three and nine weeks later, so I went to the doctor.
>
> "After one blood test, my GP [general practitioner] told me I was suffering from PCOS. I knew what it was because one of my closest friends had been diagnosed with it a couple of years ago. It was a shock, especially when my doctor told me that there was nothing I could do about it (although she did arrange for me to go for an ultrasound). She then said that the only time PCOS would be a problem was when I wanted to conceive. I was speechless. Nothing was given to me—no leaflets, no information about further reading or support groups.
>
> "So I took my health into my own hands. After reading on the Internet and buying a copy of The PCOS Diet Book, I changed my eating habits—not radically, since I'd always been pretty healthy, but I switched white flour for whole grains, ate more fruits and vegetables, and went organic as much as possible. I also snacked on nuts and dried fruit instead of chips and chocolate. And after 28 years of hardly any exercise, I went on a ten-minute jog every other day, which I quickly came to love and even look forward to!
>
> "Eight weeks after the diagnosis, I'd definitely lost weight, and my skin was clearing up, but I still hadn't gotten my period. I despaired that I'd never be able to have a baby, and I felt like a freak, not quite a woman. Another week passed—still no period. So on a whim, I bought a pregnancy test one day, and as soon as I got home, I did the test without saying a word to my partner. (Over the months leading up to the PCOS diagnosis, I'd thought I could be pregnant so many times that I felt a little like the boy who cried wolf.) To my complete surprise, the test was positive: I was pregnant!" — Jessica

I'm Pregnant! Now What?

First, you and your partner should congratulate yourselves and rejoice. Getting pregnant is a wonderful achievement, one to be proud of and excited about—especially if you've been following the PCOS fertility-boosting action plan. This has taken time and discipline, and both you and your tiny baby-to-be are reaping the health benefits already.

However, if you've had trouble getting pregnant because of PCOS, you may now feel anxious about staying pregnant. Your body didn't work the way it was supposed to when you were trying to conceive, and more than an echo of the insecurity, guilt, and worry from that time can remain with you.

It might be logical to assume that PCOS is cured or goes away when you get pregnant, but there are still no straight answers to either of these questions. "Although some women with PCOS find that their post-pregnancy cycles get more regular, there isn't any evidence that pregnancy cures PCOS," says Adam Balen. "What we do know, though, is that research does seem to indicate that a PCOS pregnancy is at greater risk." While it may feel scary to read about these facts, knowing the risks means that you can deal with them in an active and positive way.

It's been claimed that women with PCOS are generally more likely to miscarry than those without the condition.[178-9] This has been attributed to higher luteinizing hormone concentrations, which could damage egg quality, and also to the weight-management problems many women with PCOS have, since excess weight is associated with an increased risk of miscarriage.[180-1] In addition, there's also a higher rate of miscarriage for women who have become pregnant with assisted fertility treatments such as IVF.[182]

"Certainly," says Dr. Thatcher, "it appears that the risk of miscarriage is increased in mothers with PCOS, as are the risks of gestational diabetes, pregnancy-induced hypertension, unusually small or large babies, and C-sections." Some of these risks are linked to pre-pregnancy weight and others to insulin resistance, while the smaller growth rate may be specific to hormonal alterations in the PCOS ovary itself.

This all sounds alarming, but it's important to point out that early miscarriage is far more common than most realize, regardless of whether or not you have PCOS. One study in 1996 looked at 200 women who were trying to get pregnant and found a 31 percent rate of early-pregnancy loss.[183] However, once you get past weeks 12–14, other research suggests that the rate plummets to one percent and continues to fall still more as your pregnancy develops.

The first three to four weeks are vulnerable for every woman, but if you've got PCOS, there's the added worry of being at even greater risk. So what can you do to ensure that you stay pregnant and your baby-to-be is in the best health?

Your Positive Pregnancy

In this section, we've outlined what you can and should expect from your health-care provider if you have PCOS. We've also listed things you can do to help with your pregnancy, some of which are just plain common sense and good for all women, but some of which are specific to women with PCOS.

What to Expect from Your Health Service If You Have PCOS

Every pregnancy carries risk with it, regardless of your health, but do you need to see a specialist in prenatal medicine if you have PCOS? The jury is out, but most gynecologists think probably not.[184] The important thing is that you and your doctor are aware that this disorder may increase your risk of certain pregnancy-related conditions and that you're closely monitored. "Although there can be medical complications that are more common to a PCOS pregnancy, and referral to a specialist may be needed, what is most important is that your health service provides education, answers to your questions, a process to allow early identification of potential problems associated with PCOS, and care for you and your partner as individuals," says Dr. Thatcher. "There are increased risks with a PCOS pregnancy, and appropriate monitoring should be provided," agrees Adam Balen.

Pregnancy Tests

If your period is late, it makes sense to do a pregnancy test before calling your doctor, as this is probably one of the first things he or she will ask you about.

Home pregnancy tests turn positive about the time of the first missed period or 14 days after ovulation. All pregnancy tests detect levels of human chorionic gonadotropin (HCG) in your urine, resulting in a color change of a specifically designed dye indicator. HCG is produced when the fertilized embryo implants in your womb lining, and it's only present during pregnancy. Some women with PCOS say that the early hormonal changes of pregnancy often translate into fatigue, tender breasts, and frequent urination.

Further Testing in the Early Weeks

After the pregnancy test, which is usually also confirmed by a blood test, your doctor may ask you to come back in one to two weeks to test your HCG levels again. Around two weeks after ovulation, the HCG level should be 15–200 IU/L. After this, the level should double every 48 hours or so for the next two weeks (a multiple pregnancy would have a faster increase). Slower HCG increases or falling levels aren't a good sign and could suggest a possible miscarriage.

Your progesterone levels may also be measured at the same time as HCG and can help detect potential problems with the pregnancy, since progesterone is needed to sustain it. If progesterone levels aren't reassuring (under 20 pg/ml), supplemental progesterone may be recommended until about nine weeks, when the placenta is able to make all necessary progesterone by itself, and the ovaries aren't needed anymore.

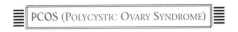

How Far Along Am I?

The typical pregnancy lasts 280 days, or 40 weeks from the last menstrual period, although if your baby is born anytime between 37 and 42 weeks, this is entirely normal.

Pregnancy is divided into three trimesters of around three months each: The first trimester is a time of rapid change and adjustment to the pregnancy; the downside is fatigue and possible morning sickness; the second trimester is usually the most enjoyable part of the pregnancy, when complications are uncommon and a woman feels that pregnant "glow"; the third can be very tiring, and as delivery day draws closer, most women have had quite enough of being pregnant.

Should I Have an Ultrasound?

Ultrasound scans at around five or six weeks are usually routine in order to date a pregnancy, but perhaps the best reason for women with PCOS to have one is for the sense of relief it can bring.[185] If there's a problem, it's probably best to find out as soon as possible to see if anything can be done.

What Should I Do If I Start Bleeding?

Call your doctor immediately, try not to panic, and get some rest. There will be bleeding in about one in three pregnancies, and about half of these will be lost, but bleeding doesn't always indicate that there's a problem. During implantation, a small amount of bleeding or spotting may occur, and it may happen again at the process of placental implantation. Generally, the greater the amount of bleeding and cramping, the greater the chance of pregnancy loss.

So what are the real risks if you're a pregnant woman with PCOS, and what can you do to ease them? Let's look at each risk factor in turn and see how you can help yourself, as well as what to expect from your doctor.

Gestational Diabetes

There haven't been any large-scale studies, but PCOS could increase the risk of gestational diabetes mellitus (GDM), defined as any degree of glucose intolerance during pregnancy. It's logical that women with PCOS, weight problems, and/or insulin resistance are at increased risk of GDM, and several small studies have suggested that around 45 percent of women with GDM have PCOS.[186]

This is one of the most common types of pregnancy complication and carries with it the risk of hypertension and cesarean section. You should be routinely screened for GDM by your health-service provider between week 24 and week 28 of your pregnancy. However, since women with PCOS and insulin resistance are known to be at higher risk, you should ensure that you're screened as early as possible.

It might also be a good idea to discuss routine testing throughout your pregnancy and after delivery. Contrary to popular belief, gestational diabetes doesn't always disappear when the baby is born—in fact, it's thought that women with GDM have a 50 percent chance of developing type 2 diabetes within 20 years of childbirth.[187]

The usual way to screen for GDM is to perform a glucose tolerance test. You'll be given a blood test after fasting the night before, and then be asked to drink some glucose-rich liquid. A second blood test will be done after an hour in order to diagnose GDM. If the test is positive, diet restrictions will be recommended, and you'll be regularly monitored.

How Is GDM Treated?

Although diabetic mothers and their babies were once at great risk, this is no longer the case, thanks to increased awareness of how to treat the condition. When blood sugar is closely controlled through diet and medication as needed, women with diabetes have normal pregnancies and healthy babies.

If you have GDM, you'll probably see your doctor more often than other expectant mothers. You'll be given more instructions, and it's crucial that you follow them. Making a diabetic pregnancy a success will take a great deal of effort on your part, but the reward—a healthy baby—will make it all worthwhile, and there may even be an upside to all this diligent self-care. One study showed that diabetic women took such good care of themselves during their pregnancies that they and their children had even fewer problems than their nondiabetic counterparts.[188]

Close vigilance is required if you have GDM. Since high glucose levels can have a harmful effect on the growing fetus, your doctor will give you strict dietary and exercise guidelines to control them. There will be more frequent appointments to check these levels, and at around 18 weeks, an ultrasound will be given to screen for fetal health. Sadly, GDM carries with it a higher risk of miscarriage, especially in the third trimester, and self-testing of fetal movement is very important. Your pregnancy will also not be allowed to progress much past 40 weeks.

There's no doubt that pregnancies with GDM are riskier, but they can also be successful. Planning is everything. Hypertension, prematurity, unexplained fetal death, and cesarean section are common complications, but these can all be avoided if you pay attention to diet and lifestyle recommendations and regular tests and checks are performed.[i]

GDM Guidelines

The key to successfully managing a diabetic pregnancy is to maintain normal blood-sugar levels. Below are components of a typical diabetic-pregnancy program designed to do just that. The instructions laid out for you by your doctor may differ slightly since they're custom-made for you (and those are the ones you should follow), but the guidelines below will give you an idea of what to expect. Whether you entered your pregnancy already diabetic or developed GDM along the way, all the following considerations will be important in working toward a safe pregnancy and healthy baby.

1. **A good diet** geared to your personal requirements should be carefully planned with your doctor. It will probably be high in complex, low-GI carbohydrates, particularly whole grains, vegetables, and beans (about half your daily diet should be from carbohydrates); moderate in protein (20–25 percent of calorie intake); and low in cholesterol and fat (30 percent of calorie intake but no more than 10 percent from saturated fat). Plenty of dietary fiber will be important (40–70 g daily are recommended), since some studies show that fiber can reduce insulin requirements in diabetic pregnancies. All this is actually pretty similar to the advice on healthful eating that a woman with PCOS should follow anyway, so if you've been following the seven-step plan from Chapter 2, you're well on your way to eating right.

As all pregnant women do, you'll probably need around 300 extra calories a day and an additional serving of protein (30 g), as well as regular healthful snacks made up of a protein and a complex-carbohydrate component (such as celery sticks and hummus), to keep your blood sugar stable. You also may need to watch the sugar content of fruit, depending on how your body handles it.

Skipping meals or snacks can dangerously lower blood-sugar levels, so be sure to eat regularly, even if morning sickness makes you feel like you don't want to. If you feel really sick, stick to bland, simple foods such as dry toast and crackers, and remember that an empty stomach will just make you feel worse. Getting sufficient calories is vital to your baby's well-being, and never try to diet during pregnancy. Weight gain should progress according to the guidelines set by your doctor, usually 25–30 pounds during the nine months. (For more on weight management in pregnancy, see page 156.)

2. **A moderate exercise program** will give you more energy and aid in regulating your blood sugar, but it must be planned in conjunction with the diet plan by your doctor. Brisk walking, swimming, and light bicycling may be suggested; and you may be asked to take some precautions, including having a snack before your workout, not allowing your heart rate to exceed 70 percent of the maximum for exercise for diabetic pregnancies, and never exercising in a warm environment.

Safe Exercise Heart Rate for Diabetic Pregnancies

To find 70 percent of the maximum safe heart rate for your age group, subtract your age from 220 and then multiply the result by .70. For example, if you're 30, you'd find it this way: 220 − 30 = 190. Then, .70 x 190 = 133.

This means that 133 beats per minute would be your safe limit of exercise intensity, which you shouldn't exceed.

3. Regular **rest and relaxation** may also be required, especially in the third trimester. If you're working outside the home, your doctor may recommend maternity leave earlier than you planned to take it, especially if your job involves standing for long periods of time or strenuous lifting.

4. In addition, you may be subject to **constant monitoring.** If your blood-sugar levels can't be controlled by diet and exercise, your doctor may recommend insulin medication. Try not to be alarmed if your health-care provider orders lots of tests for you, especially in the last three months, or even suggests hospitalization in the final weeks. This doesn't mean something is wrong, it just means that they want to make sure everything stays on track. Also, don't panic if your baby is placed in a neonatal intensive-care unit for testing immediately after delivery. This can be routine procedure for babies born to mothers with GDM.

5. Because these babies tend to be too large for full-term vaginal delivery, and because the placenta often begins to deteriorate earlier, there's a possibility of **delivery before full term**, at 38 or 39 weeks. This certainly isn't always the case though, and many women with GDM carry to full term safely.

Hypertension

Pregnant women with PCOS who are insulin resistant are also at an increased risk of hypertension or high blood pressure.[189] Hypertension is defined as a systolic pressure (top number) above 140 mm over a diastolic (bottom number) pressure over 90 mm.

Pregnancy-induced hypertension (PIH), also known as *toxemia,* is the most common medical complication. Occurring in around 8 percent of pregnancies, it's responsible for 14 percent of all maternal deaths. PIH results in constriction of the vessels of the placenta, diminishing blood flow that can restrict fetal growth.

The placenta forms the interface between mother and baby and is the site where the complications of pregnancy associated with PCOS (such as hypertension and diabetes) can manifest. It regulates the nutrient flow from mother to baby by accessing each of their needs and supplies, and plays a crucial role in pregnancy. Any damage to the placenta will damage the child.

Signs of PIH

Signs and symptoms of PIH include swelling of the hands and face with sudden weight gain due to water retention, high blood pressure (140/90 or greater in a woman who has never had high blood pressure), and protein in the urine. The condition needs to be treated immediately before it progresses to the more severe stage called *preeclampsia,* which is characterized by a further increase in blood pressure, blurred vision, and headaches. Fortunately, in women who are receiving regular medical care, the disease is invariably caught early and treated successfully, avoiding the rare outcome of it developing into full-blown eclampsia, which is characterized by convulsions and sometimes coma. Eclampsia can lead to permanent damage of the nervous system, blood vessels, and kidney in the mother, and growth retardation in the baby.

Occasionally, PIH doesn't appear until labor and delivery. It may be a reaction to stress, or it may be true eclampsia. Therefore, women who have had elevations of blood pressure in their pregnancy are watched very carefully with frequent checkups, and this is why, if you have PCOS and are therefore at a higher risk, it's worth talking about this with your doctor and making sure that you're getting the right monitoring.

Treatments for PIH

If you do have high blood pressure, your treatment will vary according to how severe the PIH is, the condition of both you and the baby, and how far along you are. With a mild case, the woman is usually hospitalized for complete bed rest (lying on the left side is best because it takes pressure off the major vessels and allows maximum blood flow to the uterus) and close observation. In some very mild cases, bed rest at home may be permitted once blood pressure has returned to a normal range. If you're allowed to stay at home, you'll be monitored by a visiting nurse and will need to make frequent visits to the doctor. It's crucial that you watch for the danger signs that can warn you that the condition is getting worse: severe headaches, visual disturbances, or upper- or mid-abdominal pain. Reducing your salt intake can also help, as can preventing excessive weight gain. Although medication may be given, beta-blockers and ACE inhibitors have been linked to fetal death, and the only safe drug for PIH is Aldomet. The best treatment, though, is delivery: In most cases, hypertension disappears once baby is delivered.

Whether in the hospital or at home, the baby's condition will be assessed regularly, and if at any point your condition worsens, or the fetus is in distress and delivery is an option, then vaginal induction of labor is the usual next step. If you have PIH, you won't be allowed to go past your due date because post term, the environment in the uterus begins to deteriorate more rapidly than usual.

Generally, the prognosis for a pregnant woman with mild PIH is good when medical care is appropriate, and pregnancy outcome is virtually the same as for a woman with normal blood pressure.

Natural Therapies for PIH

- A study by Professor Christopher Silagy and Dr. Andrew Neil reported in the *Journal of Hypertension* in 1997 showed that **garlic-powder tablets** have been proven to lower raised blood pressure.

- Hyperventilation (fast, shallow breathing), can push your blood pressure up, so learn **deep breathing exercises** and try to breathe from your abdomen.

- **Color therapy** recommends blue or indigo to lower blood pressure, so wear these colors or put up a soothing picture incorporating them.

- **Aromatherapy** uses oils of lavender, sandalwood, and rose, all of which have soothing qualities. Try them as massage oils or in a warm (not hot) bath.

- **Yoga, tai chi**, and **the Alexander Technique**, if practiced regularly, may also help lower blood pressure. Look for special pregnancy classes at your local community center.

  None of the above should be used in place of a prescription if your doctor has advised hypertensive drugs.

Obesity

As we've seen throughout the book, weight-management problems and PCOS are closely connected, and it seems that obese women with PCOS are at higher risk for complications of pregnancy when compared to obese women without this disorder. Many overweight women get pregnant and have healthy babies, but being heavier does increase the risks to mother and her baby.[190-1] These include conditions such as hypertension, diabetes, cesarean section, birth defects, blood clots, anemia, infection, more neonatal intensive care admissions, and increased risk of postnatal death in the first week.

If you have PCOS, pregnancy isn't the one time in your life when you can eat what you like and not worry about your weight. Although dieting isn't an option, you still need to keep a close eye on your body. Staying within the recommended weight gain for your height and pre-pregnancy weight is important for your baby's health and well-being, and it's important for you, too. Gaining too much now will increase your risk of GDM and PIH and make it harder for you to lose weight after the baby is born, setting you up for a long term struggle that can only make symptoms of PCOS worse. (See page 156 for our pregnancy weight-management tips.)

Big Babies, Small Babies

The average birth weight of babies born to PCOS mothers doesn't seem to differ that much from those of the general population. Infants born before 37 weeks are said to be premature, and they don't have the same risks as babies born small for their gestational age or whose growth was restricted as a result of decreased blood supply to the placenta. There can be many causes of growth restriction, but of most importance to PCOS patients are vascular problems arising from hypertension and diabetes.

Groundbreaking research by Professor David Barker at the University of Southampton, shows that what your baby weighs at birth can have a big impact on their health. There's a confirmed relationship between low birth weight and development of insulin resistance, hypertension, asthma, and type 2 diabetes. Other findings suggest that low birth weight in a girl baby predisposes her to PCOS.[192-3] This is interesting, as it would suggest that the development of PCOS has less to do with genetics, and more to do with prenatal stress, either from growth restriction, prematurity, or exposure to corticosteroids, which are used to treat individuals at risk of preterm delivery.

Babies large for their gestational age (a condition called *macrosomia*) are probably more common for women with PCOS. The major risks for these infants are related to diabetes and obesity. Gestational diabetes is uniformly associated with bigger babies, and since PCOS and diabetes are related, it's reasonable to assume that PCOS patients not only have a greater risk of GDM but also of bigger babies.[194-5] Is it possible that being large for gestational age alters fetal metabolism to such an extent that it predisposes them to later development of PCOS? Could a glucose-rich environment in the womb cause insulin resistance and/or PCOS? No studies have been done yet, but it's an interesting possibility.

Miscarriage

"I've had two miscarriages, and I'm worried about being pregnant again. My doctor tells me that it's nature's way, but that doesn't help. I'm scared: I've got PCOS, my periods are irregular, and I'm overweight. Could PCOS be a factor in my pregnancy loss? What can I do to keep from miscarrying again?" — Sue, 36 years old

The chance of a miscarriage for all pregnancies in every age group is 8–15 percent, and that rate increases to about 15–25 percent in women older than 35 and for those who have irregular menstrual cycles. Over 90 percent of miscarriages happen in the first 12 weeks, and as pregnancy progresses, the rate decreases. About 15 percent of couples trying to conceive will have three or more losses, but even after this recurrence, the chance of pregnancy is still around 70 percent.

Early losses in the first 8 weeks are most often thanks to genetic and hormonal causes and poor egg quality; between 8 and 14 weeks, they may be due to uterine abnormalities. Loss in the second trimester may be due to disorders of the placenta and sometimes chronic disease. In the third trimester, the cause is often maternal in origin and may be related to diseases of pregnancy such as diabetes and hypertension.

Is miscarriage more likely if you have PCOS? We can't say yes for sure, but one thing stands out: There are indications that women with recurring miscarriages much more often have polycystic ovaries on ultrasound.

Lesley Regan led a group that performed one of the most comprehensive studies, which reported on 2,199 women attending a recurrent-pregnancy-loss clinic in London. It found that 40 percent of the women had PCOS. Women with this condition also seem to have less viable egg quality than women without the syndrome, which can increase the risk of miscarriage.[196]

Is It My Fault?

It's important to know that except in very rare cases, such as violent trauma or drug abuse, nothing you did caused the miscarriage. All patients with impending loss are placed on bed rest, which leads many people to assume that activity increases the risk, but it doesn't. All bed rest can do is ease anxiety and avoid the guilt associated with activity. Stress may have an adverse effect on the outcome, and we'll discuss that in more detail below. Sex should be avoided since it can cause uterine contractions, but generally, once a pregnancy is established, very little can be done to alter its course.

"Losing a baby is traumatic, but don't let guilt compound your misery," says pregnancy expert Heidi Murkoff, co-author of the pregnancy bible *What to Expect When You're Expecting.* "A miscarriage is not your fault."

Will I Conceive After Miscarriage?

The chances that you'll conceive successfully again after miscarriage are good, at around 60–70 percent, even after three or four miscarriages. The risk of a second loss is only slightly higher after the first one, and a high percentage of women who miscarry during fertility treatment will go on to have a healthy baby. Pregnancy often has a positive effect on reproductive health, and some women with PCOS find that the second time around, they get pregnant easily. You shouldn't think that once fertility is impaired, it always will be. Because of the hormonal shifts involved, "pregnancy loss," says PCOS expert Dr. Thatcher, "can sometimes have a positive effect on PCOS, making the next pregnancy both easier to achieve and more likely to be successful."

"It's clear that, providing treatment is continued, the chances of a successful pregnancy are much better than even," says internationally respected infertility expert Professor Robert Winston. "Remember that a miscarriage is sure evidence that your tubes are open, that you do ovulate, and that the sperm is fertile."

When Can I Try Again?

Medically, it's probably best to wait until you've had at least one normal menstrual cycle after an early-pregnancy loss before you try again—perhaps two cycles if the loss was in the latter stages of the pregnancy.

PCOS and Breast-Feeding

There's a chance that breast-feeding may not come as easily to women with PCOS as it does to others. In a recent casual survey of mothers from two Internet PCOS support groups, 67 percent reported making enough milk, while 33 percent had an insufficient supply; of the poor-production group, 67 percent produced very little at all.

In the general population, most experts in the lactation field believe the percentage of women unable to produce sufficient milk to be less than 5 percent.

There are several different ways that PCOS could potentially interfere with lactation, although studies have yet to be done. It's well known that many PCOS sufferers are deficient in progesterone and high in androgen, and both of these can have an inhibiting effect on prolactin (the hormone crucial to milk production). Estrogen is a known inhibitor of milk production, especially in the early post-partum period, and many women with PCOS have levels that are higher than normal, so this could also potentially disrupt lactation.

Insulin also plays a vital, although less well-known, role in milk production, as women with uncontrolled diabetes mellitus won't make enough milk. Given this fact, what might be the effect of insulin resistance, which appears to be a significant factor in PCOS, upon lactation? The breast is a sensitive target organ, so if insulin can't be taken in quickly and efficiently enough, this could potentially cause lactation problems, too.

What Can I Do?

"All mothers should be aware of their community breast-feeding resources, and they should not hesitate to contact a qualified counselor if they are having problems," says Lesa Childers, international board-certified lactation consultant (IBCLC) and PCOS support chapter development coordinator, who's currently researching the link between PCOS and breast-feeding traumas. "I would strongly encourage women with PCOS to line up a professional lactation consultant in advance, and to arrange for a consultation at the first sign of possible problems. Early intervention can be very important in some cases."

Your doctor or local breast-feeding support group may be able to offer advice if things aren't going as planned—just don't be surprised if the latter seems uninformed about PCOS. Once again, making contact with other women with PCOS and breast-feeding problems via support groups or the Internet may be a source of advice and encouragement.

Sometimes trying too hard can inhibit milk production, so it's important to stop and relax once in a while, and if that means giving the baby a bottle, so be it. The "breast-feeding police" are so adamant that "breast is best" that it can leave moms who can't breast-feed or don't feel comfortable with it feeling inadequate, but every new mother needs to find what works best for her and her baby. "When breast-feeding works it is indeed a glorious experience with many benefits to mother and child," says Peggy Robin, author of *Bottlefeeding Without Guilt*, "but if it doesn't work for whatever reason there are many positive aspects of life to a bottlefeeding parent and child, which in the current climate of 'breast is best' tend to be forgotten or downplayed."

Also, keep in mind that there won't be a time in your pregnancy when you'll feel completely anxiety free, whether you have PCOS or not. That's the nature of motherhood. There's always another hurdle to face, whether it's getting pregnant, hearing the fetal heartbeat for the first time, seeing your baby move on the ultrasound screen, feeling it move in your womb, delivering a healthy baby, feeding, the first day at home, walking, talking, potty training, the first day at school, exams, first boy- or girlfriend, exams again, or their 18th birthday. You'll always worry about your kids!

Seven Steps to Boost Your Health and Well-Being During Pregnancy

What happens to you—what you eat, what you breathe, and the good and bad experiences you have—can affect your unborn baby right from the date of fertilization, when it's still too small to see with the naked eye, and for the rest of its life. Don't let this panic you, since nobody can do the right thing 100 percent of the time, but instead let it encourage you to do your best.

When you get pregnant, probably the most important things you can do are to be diligent about seeing your doctor, report anything that seems unusual, eat well, pace yourself but still get good exercise, and do everything that should be done by any pregnant woman who's determined to take good care of herself and her unborn child. Use these seven steps to a positive pregnancy as a reference to keep you on track.

Step One: Continue Eating Healthfully

As always with PCOS, get your diet and nutrition on track. Good nutrition is the key to everything in your body. Dieting during pregnancy is definitely not good, so just keep eating healthfully.

Why It's Important

Your baby's health is programmed in the womb. Researchers are learning that the developing fetus is much more sensitive to the mother's nutritional status than previously thought. Experts from St. Thomas's Hospital in London believe that the health of mothers during pregnancy affects the babies' health just as much as the life they lead as adults. Mothers who eat for two and consume a diet too high in saturated fat could be putting their unborn babies at risk for heart disease, diabetes, and high blood pressure later in life. Poor intake of one or more essential nutrients during critical periods in an organ's growth can alter the structure, size, and function of that organ, leading to the possibility of serious health consequences as they grow older.

Babies born to mothers who aren't eating properly and giving them all the nutrients they need are often born larger or smaller than they should be. The nutritional deficiencies associated with this phenomenon can have a big impact on their chances of survival after birth and their future health.[197]

Some experts believe that large-birth-weight babies (more than 8 lbs., 8 oz.) are at greater risk of developing breast cancer in later life; while babies born weighing less than 6 lbs. are more likely to be premature or stillborn, or have poor development, lowered intelligence, neurological problems, and learning difficulties. "Inadequate nutrition is associated with an increased risk of growth problems, or what is known as fetal growth restriction," says Bruce Shephard, M.D., clinical associate professor of obstetrics and gynecology at the University of South Florida College of Medicine.

There may also be a link between high-sugar diets during pregnancy and spina bifida.[198] And keep in mind that if you aren't eating well when your baby's pancreas is forming, and its size, structure, and function are affected, the child could be at greater risk of developing diabetes as an adult.

It's clear that good nutrition is vital for a healthy pregnancy and baby. But according to a 2004 survey of 1,000 women commissioned by the makers of Sanatogen ProNatal, a multivitamin supplement specially tailored to the needs of women during pregnancy, even women without PCOS don't know what to do about nutrition at this time. So what if you have this syndrome as well?

What Dietary Changes Should I Make?

If you followed a healthful diet while you were trying to conceive, such as the one in our PCOS fertility-boosting action plan, good for you. Keep going now that you're pregnant. It might also be wise to ask your doctor for pregnancy-diet information and advice and mention your increased risk of gestational diabetes at the first meeting. Even if you don't have gestational diabetes, you may want to eat a diabetic diet as a preventive measure, since it's complete and offers good nutrition.

You may be surprised to learn that if you're already eating a healthful diet before you become pregnant, you probably won't need to change it that much to cover the extra nutritional demands because your body adapts during pregnancy and becomes very efficient at absorbing and retaining nutrients. This is a time of extremes: You've never been so excited, tired, or hungry, so surely it's okay to eat a lot. After all, aren't you eating for two?

Yes, but don't go overboard. Remember, your baby-to-be is very, very tiny, not the size of the Incredible Hulk. He or she only needs an additional 300 calories a day, and that's just in the last two trimesters.

Step Two: Manage Your Weight

Excess weight has been linked with symptoms of polycystic ovaries and also to miscarriage, so weight management during pregnancy is vital for your health and the health of your baby.

In the past, when we didn't know quite so much about our bodies, gaining considerable weight may have seemed inevitable. But today, with a basic understanding of how to work with your changing body, it's possible to gain a healthy amount of weight to ensure the well-being of your baby, but also to help you reclaim your figure after the birth so that symptoms of PCOS are less likely to return. Postbaby fat is not impossible to lose if you follow some basic weight-management guidelines during and after pregnancy.

Pregnancy-Weight-Management Tips

Try to stay within the recommended range of pregnancy weight gain for your height and build because research has shown that if you do so, you're less likely to have a permanent struggle with extra pounds later.

So how much do you need to gain to satisfy your baby's needs as well as your own health? And what if you're already overweight? The Institute of Medicine in Washington, D.C., recommends a gain of 25–35 lbs. during pregnancy, and has different guidelines based on your weight and height before conception.

Pregnancy-Weight-Gain Guidelines

- If you're underweight for your height and body type (BMI less than 19.8), or if you're a teenager, the recommended total weight gain would be 28–45 lbs.

- If you're a normal weight, your recommended total gain would be 25–35 lbs.

- If you're overweight (BMI over 26), your recommended weight gain would be 20–25 lbs. (15–25 lbs. if you're obese).

- If you're expecting more than one baby, your weight gain needs to be discussed with your doctor, but it will usually be in the range of 35–45 lbs.

It's vital that all pregnant women pay attention to these guidelines, but it's particularly important if you have PCOS because being overweight during pregnancy increases the risk of miscarriage and makes post-birth weight loss more difficult, which can trigger symptoms or make them worse. So ignore all those well-meaning friends who encourage you to indulge by telling you that you're eating for two, and that this is the one time in your life when you don't have to worry about weight.

But don't restrict your intake either, even if you entered your pregnancy overweight, because dieting is definitely not a good idea. If you gain less than 20 lbs., your baby is more likely to be premature and at risk for growth problems. Babies need a constant supply of nutrients every day and can't get them all from your fat stores. If you aren't well nourished, they'll suffer, while if you gain the recommended amount of weight, you're most likely to have the healthiest weight newborn. And those born at optimal birth weight (6–8 lbs.) have the lowest risk of developmental disorders.

Around 20 lbs. of the weight you gain is for your baby's development—you don't have much control over that. Maternal fat over and above this accounts for 5–10 lbs. that prepare and strengthen your body for the demands of the growing baby. The excess fat also helps nourish both of you in the final months of pregnancy and during birth and breast-feeding. You do have control over this additional amount, but it's believed that an extra 5–10 lbs. of maternal fat increases your chances of delivering a healthy-birth-weight baby.

Why You Need to Gain Weight

There's a use for every pound you gain when you get pregnant. The weight you put on is not all for your baby, and neither is it all fat. If you were to gain 27 lbs., your weight gain would break down like this:

Baby	7.5 lbs.
Placenta	1.5 lbs.
Fat and protein stores	7.5 lbs.
Blood volume and body fluid	6 lbs.
Amniotic fluid	1.5 lbs.
Breast tissue	1 lb.
Expanded uterus	2 lbs.

How You Should Gain Weight

How you gain weight during pregnancy is almost as important as how much weight you gain:

— During **the first three months**, you should ideally be gaining between one and four pounds. You don't need to eat more than you normally do at this time; you just need to make sure that your diet is healthy and nutritious. Your doctor or midwife will also give you a diet plan with recommended amounts of proteins, carbohydrates, fats, and other pregnancy food guidelines.

— **From three to six months**, it's the optimal time for you to gain weight. Your baby needs an increased food intake, so you should be eating an additional 300 calories each day. These should come from healthy, nutritious food choices such as a sandwich on whole-grain bread and a glass of milk. Weight gain at this time should be at a steady rate of one to two pounds a week.

— **From six to eight months**, you should continue to gain about a pound a week, with weight loss slowing in the ninth month. While the second trimester is a time of rapid weight gain, the third trimester is a time for slowing down, conserving your energy, and preparing for the baby.

Although these guidelines sound very specific, they're just to show you that there's a reason behind even a small increase in weight, and it will help you and your baby-to-be. But remember: Excess weight isn't an inevitable consequence of pregnancy for women with PCOS. Everyone is unique, and it may be impossible to rigorously stick to these guidelines; such an approach could increase your stress levels and be detrimental to both you and your baby. There will be times when you gain more than others; and morning sickness, fluid retention, and food cravings can all cause fluctuations. Keeping an idea of what to aim for, however, can alert you to potential problems (change that's too slow or too fast can be early warning signs) and help you avoid overeating and gaining too much.

Step Three: Get Rid of Unhealthy Habits

Avoid cigarettes, alcohol, and caffeine. You don't need anything that could compromise your pregnancy or make symptoms of PCOS worse.

Smoking

Smoking suppresses your appetite, robs your baby-to-be of vital nutrients, and can interfere with your ability to eat enough food. You also increase the risk of miscarriage, preterm delivery, and a low-birth-weight baby. You'd have to be foolish not to acknowledge the harmful effects smoking can have on a developing fetus. Pregnancy is a time for new beginnings, and what better time for you to quit this dangerous and harmful habit, for both your health and the health of your child?

If you smoke and want to quit, talk to your doctor. Starting an exercise program will help with weight management, and be sure to take a multivitamin, too. There are many ways to give up smoking, but perhaps the most effective is to simply stop. The nicotine will pass out of your system within a few days, so when you crave a cigarette after that, you aren't craving nicotine, but the habits you associated with it. What you have to do now is try to find other habits to replace smoking. With a baby coming into your life, this shouldn't be too hard. There are a million things for you to think about and do—you haven't got time for cigarettes anymore!

Alcohol

Any alcohol that you drink during pregnancy is passed through the placenta into the baby's bloodstream. No one is really quite sure what the safe limit is, so it's best to avoid it altogether and make your own fresh juices, milkshakes, and sparkling mineral water drinks instead. Even beers and wines that claim to be alcohol free or low in alcohol may have harmful additives and chemicals that can have unknown effects on your unborn child's health.

Babies born to heavy drinkers can have what's known as *fetal alcohol syndrome* where growth and intelligence are affected. Even a moderate amount may be harmful. All pregnant women are advised not to drink. If you enjoy alcohol, talk to your doctor.

Caffeine

Caffeine is a central-nervous-system stimulant, but so far, no study has proved conclusively that it can cause low-birth-weight babies. We do know that caffeine withdrawal can affect newborns and cause feeding difficulties, colic, and irritability. Because of the uncertainty concerning how harmful caffeine is, it's probably wise to keep your consumption down—say, no more than two cups of coffee a day.

Illegal Drugs

All drugs are dangerous for your baby-to-be. Within 30 minutes of ingestion or injection, they're in the fetal blood, too. Just don't take them. If you do have an addiction or dependency problem, talk to your doctor immediately.

Medications

All pharmaceuticals, whether over the counter or from your doctor, are potentially harmful during pregnancy. Always discuss with your health-care provider any medications, painkillers, or dietary supplements you're taking in order to ensure that they're safe to use.

Unsafe Food

Foods to avoid during your pregnancy include junk food, caffeine, dishes that have been fried or highly seasoned, and rare or under-cooked meat, poultry, and shellfish. Especially avoid raw eggs, raw meat, and unpasteurized foods like soft goat cheese and mold-ripened cheeses, such as brie and blue cheese, which may have been infected by harmful organisms. Cottage cheese and hard cheeses, however, are fine. The U.K.'s Food Standards Agency also recently advised pregnant women to avoid entirely mercury-contaminated fish such as tuna, swordfish, shark, and marlin. Grilling can produce harmful substances in meat, so avoid this method of cooking.

But Don't Be a Saint!

Just because you're pregnant doesn't mean that you have to become a food saint. If you enjoy chocolate, ice cream, and other naughty food choices that are high in fat and sugar, go ahead and eat them. If about 90 percent of your diet is healthy and nutritious, you can afford to spoil yourself once in a while. A balanced diet contains a wide variety of foods, and even chocolate contains antioxidants that are now thought to be good for you. Just don't go overboard, and you can enjoy a little of everything in moderation: one bar of chocolate, not five, or one scoop of ice cream, not the whole container.

Step Four: Exercise Regularly and Gently

We've seen how important regular exercise is if you have PCOS, especially as part of your fertility-boosting action plan. It's also significant after you get pregnant.[199] You may think that there's no conclusive evidence showing that exercise improves the health of your unborn child, and you'll probably feel too tired. You may worry that physical changes will make it difficult for you to move, bend, and even breathe; and you're going to gain weight anyway—so why bother keeping fit when you're pregnant?

Why Exercise During Pregnancy?

- It keeps your muscles, bones, and heart strong.

- It stimulates your metabolism so that you burn calories faster, which helps you maintain a healthy weight throughout the nine months.

- It improves your sense of physical and emotional well-being by helping relieve backaches and preventing morning sickness, varicose veins, and constipation; as well as lifting your spirits and easing stress.

- It makes it easier for you to get fit and slim again afterward—vital if you've got PCOS—and to be an active caregiver for your child.

- There's evidence that exercise during pregnancy can reduce the risk of diabetes, which women with PCOS are at an increased risk of.

If you took a nine-month break from any type of exercise, you'd be much less fit afterward, and it would take quite a while to get your form back. Although you won't be able to train vigorously, you can still maintain your fitness levels—or even boost them—so that returning to normal activity afterward is a smoother transition, which will be better for your health, your child, your relationship, social life, and career. You'll also be maintaining the healthy habit of exercise as a PCOS-fighting tool to help keep any symptoms under control once you've given birth. If you didn't exercise before, then this isn't a good time to start a strenuous program; but on the other hand, pregnancy is no reason to put off being active.

Is Exercise Safe During Pregnancy?

During the dark days when having a baby was considered an illness, you weren't supposed to exercise. Now we know better, and the American College of Obstetricians and Gynecologists encourages expectant mothers to keep active because it seems to be good for you and your baby.

The only way you put your baby-to-be in danger is if your activity is exhausting, strenuous, and violent, such as running a marathon or climbing a mountain. But moderate activity in a healthy, well-nourished expectant mother can actually prevent health problems such as excessive weight gain, poor posture, back pain, and poor body image, something many of us with PCOS have enough trouble with as it is.

As long as you don't have any obstetric or medical complications, including those listed in this section, you can continue to exercise and derive benefits from it. If you've already achieved cardiovascular fitness, you should be able to safely maintain that level throughout pregnancy and the postpartum period.

Always seek advice before doing any exercise if you suffer, or have suffered in the past, from any of these conditions:

- Pregnancy-induced hypertension

- Preterm rupture of the amniotic sac and leaking of amniotic fluid

- Preterm labor during a prior or the current pregnancy, or both

- Incompetent cervix cerclage (the procedure by which the cervix is stitched closed after conception to prevent it from opening early)

- Persistent second or third trimester bleeding

- Intrauterine growth retardation (inadequate development of the fetus or placenta)

- A history of miscarriage in the first trimester

There isn't any research proving that fit women have easier pregnancies and deliveries, but many doctors feel that fitness helps women cope better. In the words of Dr. Arlene Jacobs, obstetrician and gynecologist at the Medical Center of Plano in Texas, "It is safe to exercise when you are pregnant. For all pregnant women, especially women with PCOS, I recommend regular exercise. I'd only have reservations if a woman has never exercised before. She must start very gradually and slowly."

However, do consult your doctor before you begin any program. It's also wise to discuss continuing any exercising you were doing before you got pregnant. Your health-care practitioner will be able to talk to you about any medical circumstances that might have an impact on your workouts. Certain conditions, such as those listed above, may require you to modify your exercise program or to avoid it altogether.

Fit to Be a Mom

You may feel that simply being pregnant is enough of a workout, and you'd rather rest than go for a walk or a jog. That's fine— you don't have to exercise when you are pregnant. It's just that regular exercise will help manage your weight and strengthen your body for the demands of pregnancy, childbirth, and postpartum recovery.

Try to think of these nine months as a training period: You're training to have a baby and be a fit mom. You don't want to be listless, stiff, and out of shape when your baby arrives. One of the greatest gifts you can give your child is being fit and alert enough to welcome him or her into the world with energy.

Step Five: Reduce Stress

We've seen how damaging stress can be if you have PCOS, and how it can negatively impact your fertility; not surprisingly, it isn't good when you're pregnant, either. There's a wealth of international research from America, Ireland, Spain, France, Australia, and Britain suggesting that babies are aware of their mother's emotions while they're in the womb: A relatively calm pregnancy tends to produce calmer babies, and a stressful life can affect a baby's neurological system for good.[200] This may have many different potential effects, ranging from an impaired ability to deal with stress to hormonal disorders like PCOS.

Stress also isn't good news if you're undergoing fertility treatment. A study published in March 2004 suggests that psychological and relationship problems cause many couples to stop treatment. Researchers in Sweden surveyed 974 couples who were having IVF, and writing in the journal *Fertility and Sterility,* they said that 26 percent of the group dropped out for psychological reasons, while 15 percent were having marital problems.

Cut down on stress in all areas of your life. Make room for your pregnancy, and don't just keep going forward regardless of your own well-being. Instead, take time to consciously relax for a minimum of 20 minutes every day, and as you do, visualize your baby safe, secure, and happy in your womb.

Communicate with Your Baby

International research suggests that spoken and unspoken (happy thoughts) communication between a mother and unborn baby can begin as early as the first few days after conception. Why not take a few moments each day to do a simple visualization exercise such as this one?

Close your eyes, breathe deeply, and in your mind's eye, see your baby nestling safely in your womb lining and staying there, growing, safe, and secure. Send messages of love, happiness, and welcome, telling it that it's safe, loved, and wanted. And if you or your partner talk out loud or play calming, uplifting music (Mozart is often recommended) to your unborn child, prenatal research from Ireland suggests your baby can hear as early as 17 weeks, even though the actual ears don't form until week 33.

Mother Yourself

Take some time for yourself. This can be an amazing opportunity to learn the importance of self-nurturing and plant the roots of self-love so deep that after giving birth, you'll be able to replenish yourself and give authentically to your child without losing your identity.

"Every woman not only richly deserves self-care," says Jennifer Louden, author of the best-selling *Woman's Comfort Book,* "but she must have it if she is to survive and thrive as a mother. Pregnancy offers us the excuse to be gentle on ourselves. That excuse can become a habit. That habit can slowly become a lovingly held belief: 'I am worth self-care, not just when I am carrying a child, but every day.'"

Although you probably feel as if all your time and attention should go to your growing baby, some must be given to you, too. Many mothers say that they wish they'd taken advantage of their pregnancy more. For some reason, it didn't dawn on them that this might be the last time in quite a while that they could take it easy. So repeat to yourself over and over again: *Enjoy this time. Slow down and relax because it may never come again.* Of course, you want to keep your baby's welfare firmly in mind, but it's vital for you also to emphasize your needs.

Mothering yourself and reducing stress means taking time for yourself and doing what makes you feel good. Sometimes in the flurry of our responsibilities, we forget how to make this happen. Use the suggestions below as starting points for weaving relaxation and enjoyment into your life.

1. **Let go of the "shoulds"**: Every time you catch yourself saying or thinking *I should do that,* try changing the *should* into a *could* to see if that helps reduce feelings of stress.

2. Try taking a mini relaxation break every time you need to use the restroom. **Make relaxation a habit** because it prepares you for labor, when knowing how to relax can help you in a big way. When you sit down, consciously relax your shoulders and jaw. Close your eyes and breathe deeply (hopefully the restroom will be clean!), and silently say a calming word to yourself (for example, *peace, love,* or *chocolate*). Then exhale through your mouth and repeat several times.

3. When you feel conflicted, stressed, and unable to relax, **indulge in some positive self-talk.** Many inner voices are critical or negative, but pregnancy provides a unique inner voice that can calm you and remind you of what's important. Find a few moments when you can be alone, then close your eyes and concentrate on breathing deeply, feeling the breath going down into your belly. After a minute or two, let any thought that occurs to you come into your mind. It might be *Why can't I relax?* or it could simply be *Good morning.* Now relax and let the energy of your pregnancy answer your question. Don't strain; just tune in. You'll almost certainly get a "be good to yourself" answer. Try it and see.

Positive Self-Talk

Here are some possible thoughts and responses:

- *I feel stressed.* Breathe. Take it easy and feel the new life inside you.

- *I feel so tired.* Take some time out and focus on the beginning of this journey.

- *I'm afraid.* Don't pressure yourself to feel happy all the time. Find what makes you feel good and stop worrying about what you should and shouldn't do.

Finally, if you really can't relax, allow yourself to be good to your unborn child. Motivate yourself by saying, *My baby needs me to sit down or relax or be good to myself.* After you get used to this, try again to transfer this caring behavior to yourself. Visualize how connected you are to your baby, and feel in your heart that caring for and loving this tiny being can't be separated from looking after yourself. When you take your prenatal vitamins, whisper some positive thoughts to yourself, such as *I feel honored and special to be a mother.*

4. **Remind yourself of your achievements:** Every time you feel your baby kick, think of all the times in your life when you've felt proud of yourself. Small achievements count just as much as big ones, and the events you recall don't have to be connected to your pregnancy.

5. When you walk or use the stairs, remind yourself that your body is keeping two people alive. **Praise your body**, and congratulate yourself on keeping active.

6. After each prenatal appointment, **do something special for yourself.** Perhaps you'd like a pedicure or to spend a few hours browsing in your local bookstore. It doesn't matter what it is, as long as it makes you feel good.

7. Buy a special notebook and pen and **keep a journal of pregnancy.** Record your hopes, fears, thoughts, and dreams. This time is ripe with insight, so write down what you want to when you want to. It will calm you and help you celebrate and make sense of your experience.

8. Pregnancy offers a unique opportunity to **create or strengthen your support team** so that it's in place postpartum for when you really need it. When you're pregnant, you'll find that it's easy to connect with other women and make new friends. New moms, loving friends, an understanding family, and of course, an understanding doctor and midwife are essential for your medical, physical, and emotional health, both during and after pregnancy. Allow your team to nurture and support you. People who care about you are generally really happy to listen, hug, reassure, or lend a helping hand so that you can put your feet up and relax.

Step Six: Check Out Complementary Therapies

Perhaps you've used complementary therapies to help treat symptoms of PCOS or to increase your chances of getting pregnant.

You might like to think about continuing some of these after you conceive. You may experience a host of uncomfortable physical symptoms, from hemorrhoids to heartburn, and just when you need them the most, conventional drugs are off-limits. Even taking aspirin is no longer a safe option. Yet help *is* available, say fans of complementary medicine. Natural therapies offer some of the safest, and often only, ways to get relief.

Morning Sickness and Nausea

Laura, age 37, felt so nauseated during her second pregnancy that she couldn't leave home for fear she'd faint. *"The doctor could only prescribe bed rest, but that wasn't an option with a 14-month-old to look after,"* she says. A friend persuaded her to visit a naturopath. *"Within days of following the naturopath's advice to take regular vitamin and mineral supplements, drink lots of dried ginger root tea, and press acupressure points at the base of my wrist, I felt better."*

Terrible feelings of sickness and nausea are thought to affect over 80 percent of pregnant women in some way. Doctors can't offer any approved pharmaceutical treatment, but research shows that natural therapies may offer relief.

A study reported in the *Archives of Gynecology and Obstetrics* talked about a significant reduction in nausea and vomiting in women who took vitamin and mineral supplements; a study of 30 women suffering from nausea who took part in trials recorded in the *European Journal of Obstetrics & Gynecology and Reproductive Biology* found relief from taking 250 mg of ginger in capsule form four times a day; and in the *Journal of the Royal Society of Medicine*, at least seven randomized trials of acupressure and acupuncture for pregnancy sickness concluded that these treatments can work.

Complementary Therapies and PCOS Pregnancy

"Most of the pregnant women I treat have been to their doctors first," says homeopath, nurse, and prenatal teacher Anna Foxell, who works with expectant mothers in London. "They have been down the conventional road, and it hasn't helped them. Pregnancy is the ideal time to discover the benefits of alternative therapies, not only because drugs are off-limits, but also because when a woman is pregnant she tends to be more open to new things. I've found that the cure rate during pregnancy is much higher. You have to drop your defenses in order to unconditionally love a child."

But are complementary therapies safe during pregnancy if you've got PCOS? On the whole, natural therapies can't harm you or your baby-to-be, but problems can arise when alternative practitioners unknowingly give pregnant women with PCOS the wrong herb, dose, or advice, so do your research. These options can be wonderfully useful if you take them with caution and under supervision from your health-care practitioner and/or pharmacist and always read the labels.

More and more experts are taking this view, including Dr. Tanvir Jamil, co-author of *The Alternative Pregnancy Handbook* and a practicing GP with specialist knowledge of complementary medicine; and obstetrician Yehudi Gordon, who founded the Hospital of St. John and St. Elizabeth's Birth Unit in 1981, where midwives and obstetricians recommend, in addition to conventional care, a network of complementary therapists, including osteopaths, ayurvedic practitioners, homeopaths, aromatherapists, nutritionists, acupuncturists, and self-hypnosis therapists.

"We view these therapies as extremely powerful aids for pregnancy, labor, and postnatal health," says Gordon.

Treatments to Avoid

Certain herbs, essential oils, and nutritional supplements can be as potentially harmful as drugs during pregnancy—tansy, sage, and large doses of vitamin A, to name just a few—and normally safe therapies can be extremely dangerous. For example, naturopathic treatments that include fasting, going on a restricted diet, or even drinking lots of water to relieve heartburn and flush out toxins (since the fetus needs a steady supply of nutrients, more than two quarts of water a day can overburden the kidneys). Hydrotherapy, which involves alternating hot and cold baths, can promote healing, but raising body temperature above 100.4°F isn't recommended for women expecting a baby. Some traditional ayurvedic medicines may contain mercury and lead, which are dangerous during pregnancy. Yoga, massage, and acupuncture can relieve stress, but only in the hands of practitioners skilled in the treatment of pregnant women.

Alternative therapies shouldn't be used carelessly at any time, especially when you're pregnant. "Natural" doesn't always mean "safe." Conventional pharmaceuticals and treatments must undergo rigorous clinical trials to demonstrate safety before being licensed as medicine, but the majority of herbal remedies and alternative therapies are exempt. How can a pregnant woman know her choices are safe? She should check with her doctor and make sure she works with a qualified practitioner of alternative medicine. Paula Marie from the British Complementary Medicine Association cautions, "There should be no treatment at all in the first three months, during labor and ten days after, and no physical therapies, like massage, from the seventh month."

Complementary therapies may help you stay well and have a smoother, calmer pregnancy and labor, but always check first with your doctor and your complementary practitioner to ensure safety. The following treatments have been recommended and used during pregnancy by women with PCOS.

1. **Acupuncture and acupressure** can be used to treat numerous problems in pregnancy, such as aches and pains, morning sickness, and headaches. It's safe to use during pregnancy and breast-feeding and brings relief to pain that's unresponsive to conventional therapy, thus enabling a decreased use of painkilling drugs. You'll feel relaxed afterward, and it works well with conventional therapy.

2. **Alexander technique**, with its emphasis on correct posture, is excellent for almost all aspects of pregnancy, especially back pain, pelvic-floor strengthening, fatigue, stress, anxiety, low moods, and headaches. There are plenty of local courses available where you can learn the technique and eventually practice it by yourself without the presence of a teacher. The exercises should be done twice daily for 10 to 15 minutes.

3. **Kinesiology** is a system of manipulation and massage that can be particularly useful for backaches, neck pain, stiffness, fatigue, and depression. It's excellent for helping aches and pains during pregnancy and after giving birth.

4. **Aromatherapy** is now so popular for pregnancy and labor that many midwives often include its use in their advice for prenatal classes. Some also practice aromatherapy themselves and will use it to help you make childbirth a positive experience. The basics are easily self-taught from books or local courses, but do bear in mind that there are certain essential oils you can't use at all during pregnancy (such as sage, clove, cinnamon, fennel, and tarragon) and some you shouldn't use in the first trimester (rosemary and peppermint, for example). Always make sure you check for contraindications.

5. The following **Bach Flower Remedies** are suitable for symptoms in pregnancy:

- *Rescue remedy* for emotional and physical stress

- *Olive* for tiredness

- *Crab apple* for morning sickness

- *Aspen* for anxiety

- *Mimulus, walnut,* or *rock rose* for fear

- *Mustard* for depression

These remedies are simple to use at home and are widely available from health-food stores.

6. **Herbal medicine** can help alleviate many of the uncomfortable symptoms of pregnancy. You may want to try one of these:

- *Ginger* and *chamomile* for morning sickness

- *Lime flower* for stress

- *Peppermint* for indigestion

- *Psyllium seeds* for constipation

- *Yarrow tea* or *cranberry juice* for cystitis (bladder infections)

Herbal medicine is safe, if prescribed by a professional herbalist, and has few side effects. Do make sure, though, that if you've been taking any herbal supplements prior to getting pregnant, you discontinue them until you've checked their safety with your doctor and a qualified herbalist.

7. **Homeopathy** is very safe and can help a lot of pregnancy-related symptoms, and there are very few side effects. To get the maximum benefit, make sure that you see a qualified homeopath experienced in treating pregnant woman before self-prescribing.

8. Many women find **hypnotherapy** helpful. It can ease stress, morning sickness, pain, and mild depression; and it can also help increase your confidence and change unwanted bad habits, such as swearing and smoking. It's easily taught and good practitioners are readily available.

9. **Massage** is one of the best therapies to use during pregnancy because it's safe, little equipment is required, and expectant moms often experience positive feelings and a sense of calm during and

after the treatment. However, as with all physical therapies, it shouldn't be used after the seventh month.

10. **Meditation** will help keep you healthy and happy if you practice for around 10 to 20 minutes every day. It's easy to learn and do, and can be used for specific ailments such as nausea, stress, high blood pressure, fatigue, and depression.

11. The advantage of **naturopathy** is that it's safe during pregnancy. Common-sense diet and lifestyle changes, such as those we discussed earlier in this chapter, will be recommended to support the health of you and your child. If you've been taking any nutritional supplements or it's suggested that you do, check with your doctor to see if they're safe at this time.

12. **Reflexology** can be particularly helpful for a whole host of pregnancy-related symptoms such as headaches, nausea, anxiety, constipation, and other aches and pains. It's gentle, calming, and relaxing.

We've listed the therapies most suitable for women with PCOS, but there are many other complementary therapies that are now commonly used during pregnancy. These include **yoga, tai chi, color therapy, Rolfing, shiatsu, osteopathy, chiropractic, ayurveda,** and **autogenic therapy.** (For more information on all of the above complementary therapies, see our Resource Guide.)

Step Seven: Listen to Your Body

As long as you don't go to extremes, there's no evidence to suggest that work, exercise, or travel have an adverse effect on pregnancy. Stress is a big danger, but you can find ways to deal with that. Pregnancy isn't an illness, and although you may find it harder to get around, you can do a lot of the same things that you normally did.

Don't Push Yourself

If you're worried that you might do something to endanger your baby, stop where you are and don't push. This may mean taking some time off work, dropping a commitment, or changing your routine. Above all, *listen to your body.* It will tell you when you aren't taking care of yourself. If you're tired, rest; if you're hungry, eat; and if you feel stiff, take some time to stretch.

If you're worried about anything, talk to your doctor, and if you think you could have a problem, get it evaluated. In the past, you may have been able to just struggle on, regardless of PCOS symptoms flaring up or feeling unwell, but you simply can't do that now. Life isn't just about you anymore—it's about you and your future child.

In trying to have a successful pregnancy, it's easy to lose sight of the object of all this planning and attention. Becoming a mom is both exciting and daunting, but try to remember that from now on your child relies on you for love, security, and the best that you can give.

After the Birth

Don't forget that taking good care of yourself by eating well, exercising regularly, managing your weight, and watching your stress levels are just as important now as they were before and during pregnancy.

Keep on Eating Well

A healthful diet is extremely important after you've given birth. "The baby more or less 'vacuum cleans' the mother in terms of nutrients, [while] in the womb and breast-feeding," says nutrition expert Oscar Umahro Cadogan, who is a lecturer for the Danish Institute of Optimal Nutrition. Umahro urges all new mothers to make sure that they continue to eat healthfully once the baby is born, not just because a breast-feeding baby's health and well-being depends on proper nutrition, but because yours do, too.

The fact is that many women get completely run down by pregnancy and breast-feeding. It's important that once the baby is born, or when you've stopped breast-feeding, that you continue eating healthfully. If you have PCOS, good nutrition and managing your weight are just as important now as they've always been. Be especially careful to eat well in the first six months postpartum in order to take advantage of the "weight-loss window" (discussed below). And after that, keep on eating healthfully (according to the guidelines we gave in Chapter 2) to help manage your symptoms.

Keep Active, Too

Exercise may be the last thing on your mind with a new baby to care for 24 hours a day, but it really is crucial for weight management and improving your health and well-being. In the first few weeks, gentle walking is enough, but once you've had your six-week checkup, and the doctor is happy with your progress, there's no reason why you shouldn't gradually increase your exercise levels so that you're exercising for 30 minutes or more four or five times a week.

Bye-Bye Baby Fat

The first six months after birth is your weight-loss opportunity. Research into postpartum hormonal changes reveals exciting news for women with PCOS: At no other time in your life is your body so efficient at weight loss, and at no other time is there such an opportunity for you to override your *set point,* the place your body always seems to return to after you lose weight. You could even end up weighing less than before you got pregnant.[201-2]

In the first few postpartum months, your body is primed for weight loss. During this time, your fat-burning, appetite-suppressing hormones are activated. Normally, your internal chemistry favors weight gain, as every woman with PCOS who's tried to lose weight knows all too well. But now, for around six months, things are very different. When you give birth, estrogen and progesterone levels plummet, but your metabolism remains high. It takes an average of four to six months for your hormones to get back to their pre-pregnancy state (longer if you're breast-feeding), and this time of hormonal adjustment gives you a unique chance to lose weight and perhaps revise your body's set point.

How do you take advantage of this? Remember that things are different now: You're primed for weight loss and searching for balance, so you don't need to diet or restrict your food intake drastically. All you need to do is relax and eat a healthful, nutritious diet, such as the one we outlined in our PCOS fertility-boosting plan. There are a couple points to remember, though:

1. **Crash dieting is a mistake** since it will simply confuse your metabolism. It could trigger a starvation response that makes you cling to fat and sets you up for long-term problems. You may feel uncomfortable with the extra weight you gained during pregnancy and want to lose it all as quickly as you can, but dieting and vigorous exercise right now are the worst things you can do. Just eat healthfully, exercise gently, be patient for a few months, and let your body do the rest.

Many women with PCOS who eat well during the postpartum period find that weight management is less of a problem after giving birth than it was before they got pregnant. Former Spice Girl Victoria Beckham was diagnosed with PCOS in her teens, and her svelte postbaby figure is a celebrity example of success.

If your weight is under control, you're less likely to get as many PCOS symptoms. Could this be the reason some people claim that having a baby cures PCOS? The six-month weight-loss window could be the reason why their symptoms don't return to the same extent after having a baby.

2. Of course, you'll wonder **how you can expect to lose the weight.** Typically, after delivery, you can expect to lose around 12 lbs. This isn't the 20 lbs. or so you may have hoped for, but don't worry—in the weeks that follow you'll continue to lose weight gradually if you just choose simple, nutritious foods and get your body moving with gentle walking. This will encourage you to lose weight as naturally and as quickly as possible.

In the next six weeks, you'll enter another round of weight loss and will usually lose an additional 9–12 lbs. After that, any weight loss is baby fat (it won't fall off automatically, and it's up to you to gently work it off), but remember that for up to six months postpartum, your hormones are still working in your favor, so as long as you keep eating well and exercising gently, the weight will melt away.

This isn't always easy with a new baby to care for, but your health and well-being should be just as important now as your child's. Perhaps you could ask a friend or relative to look after the baby for an hour or so in order to shop for some healthful foods. Or perhaps you could take your baby for a walk every day to ensure that you get some gentle exercise.

After six months—usually around the time your periods and/or symptoms of PCOS return—your hormones will settle down into their usual patterns, and it won't be as easy to lose weight. Don't panic, however, if after six or seven months you still haven't lost all the weight, because you have an opportunity to rethink your approach to body image and weight loss. You have a new baby, a new body, and a new life—so forget the old rules.

In your new life as a mother, you won't diet anymore. Dieting belongs to the past, so now you'll eat healthful, nutritious foods that are good for you. You'll keep active to encourage your body to be fit and healthy, and most important, you'll keep a sense of perspective and enjoy the way you look.

Make Sure You Support and Take Time for Yourself

Looking after a new baby is stressful and lonely at times, and you'll need all the support you can get from your partner, your friends, and your family members. It's especially important for you and your partner to share the child care and be involved in each other's lives and feelings. Don't just divert all your energy to the baby.

Finally, remember the advice about mothering yourself that we gave earlier. Try to carve out some time for yourself every day, because a new baby can be all-consuming, but you also need to find some time for you. This can be as simple as a relaxing bath at the end of the day or doing something else that you enjoy, such as reading a book, listening to music, or spending time with friends when your baby naps.

You could also ask a friend or family member you trust to look after your baby for a few hours while you go out for a meal with your partner, get some exercise, go shopping, indulge in a massage, or simply have some time alone. Yes, there may be 101 things on your housework and baby "to do" list, and it may seem indulgent to spend time on yourself, but always remember that the greatest gift you can give your child is a healthy, happy, and relaxed mom.

Good luck! Here's to your child of the future: May he or she be healthy and happy and bring you much joy.

Chapter Seven

Riding the PCOS Emotional Roller Coaster: Staying Sane and Happy Throughout Your Fertility Journey

Worrying about whether you should—or indeed, can—have a child may bring up a whole range of emotions including anxiety, despair, anger, and depression, as well as delight, excitement, and joy.

> *"I remember the first time that I saw infertility and PCOS marked as my diagnosis. I thought it couldn't apply to me—but as each failed cycle went by, I was forced to realize that yes, I had PCOS, and I might be infertile. It was a strange condition to accept when I'd always imagined myself with at least three kids, yet the reality of being able to do so now seemed beyond me."*
> — Ann, 29 years old

If anxiety about your fertility is making you feel confused and vulnerable, or if you're undergoing fertility treatment and finding the whole experience traumatic and invasive, keep reading for positive ideas about how to cope with the emotional roller coaster. There are three main areas that bring about their own peculiar set of ups and downs when you have PCOS and you're tackling the issue of fertility.

Area One: Biological-Clock Anxiety—Magnified!

The phenomenon of biological-clock anxiety is a fairly new trend, since women put off having children for much longer than they did a generation ago. But with PCOS, the effect of wondering about the right time to have a baby is intensified by worries about how long it might take to get pregnant.

Previously, medical experts had thought that a woman's fertility started to decline in her 30s, but findings from researchers at the University of Padua in Italy and the National Institute of Environmental Health Sciences in North Carolina suggest that a woman may start to find it harder to conceive in her late 20s. And according to fertility experts at Utrecht University in Holland, women who delay having children for career reasons should be told how falling fertility levels could hamper their chances of having a baby later in life.

What happens if you're diagnosed with PCOS and are suddenly faced with the prospect of fertility problems? The fear of being robbed of any choice regarding motherhood can often prompt women with PCOS to make decisions much earlier than they would have liked.

If you have PCOS, there's no escaping the fact that by the age of 35 (at the latest) you really do need to confront the issue of whether or not you want children. But what if you really don't know? There are tools and techniques recommended by experts to help women cope with biological-clock anxiety. For example, talking to women who have chosen not to become mothers can be very helpful in offering insights into the consequences of that choice. Spending time with children to see what you'd be letting yourself in for can also be useful. But although they may help, none of these techniques can answer the most important question: *How much do I really want a child?* If you're almost ready to make a decision, there are definitely some things you should be asking yourself.

Questions to Ask Yourself about Becoming a Mother

- Am I prepared for the possible discomfort associated with pregnancy and childbirth?

- Am I willing to open up my relationship or marriage to a third party (the child)?

- Am I prepared to devote the first few months of my baby's life entirely to him or her?

- Am I prepared to feel lonely and isolated at times?

- If I plan to raise my baby alone, am I prepared to endure criticism, and am I willing to accept that it will be harder for me to find a partner after the baby is born?

- Am I willing to embrace the chaos a child brings: the sleepless nights and the loss of free time, routines, control, and personal space?

- Am I prepared for the overwhelming responsibility of motherhood?

- Have I thought about the negative possibilities as well as the positive: That is, what if my baby has health problems, my partner leaves, and I lose my job?

- Am I prepared to love my child whatever its sex, temperament, and personality—and not just as a baby, but also as a child, teenager, and young adult?

- Am I prepared for the cost and extra expense a child can bring? If I'm going to continue working, am I prepared for the stresses of juggling home and career?

If you don't feel ready, your lifestyle isn't conducive to having a baby, or you're not really sure you want to do this, it makes sense to wait, even though PCOS and declining fertility may be urging you to make up your mind. Talking to trusted friends, your partner, and loved ones, or seeing a counselor or therapist can be helpful. It's also well worth investigating the issue with other women in a PCOS support group or specific biological-clock-anxiety support groups, such as those run by RESOLVE in the U.S.

What about Waiting?

The idea of having children can often override whether or not you actually want to have them and will be a good mother. The purpose of therapy, counseling, support groups, or talking things through with an understanding friend or family member isn't for you to resolve all your emotional conflicts, but to help you decide what you really want so that PCOS or other people don't pressure you into making a decision.

Giving yourself permission to wait does carry the risk that you may not be able to have a child in the future—if this happens, regret and sadness are inevitable, but always remember that there were reasons for the choices you made. And as we'll discuss in the next chapter, there are other ways to bring children into your life, such as adopting, fostering, or mentoring. There's so much emphasis on pregnancy and giving birth that it overshadows the fact that it's what happens to children *after they're born* that really matters.

Ambivalence about Motherhood

As you explore these issues, you may even find that motherhood isn't for you after all. Deciding not to have children involves coping with the inevitable fear of regretting your decision later in life, although you can also think of all the energy, time, freedom, experiences, and extra money you'll have. Remember that mothers have their regrets and frustrations, too—no life choice is perfect. There's no reason why a woman without children should feel alone. In fact, the number of women remaining childless by choice is increasing. According to the U.S. census, nearly 20 percent of women in the baby-boomer generation aren't having children. America now has a child-free network with more than 50 meeting places for couples without kids. The organization believes that we all should be respected for who we are and not be judged by whether or not we have children. Such a life can be full, productive, and happy and should be carefully considered if you feel ambivalent about children. In the U.K., the charity Issue has set up an organization called More to Life, an exciting new development that aims to build a network of support across the U.K. for the growing number of child-free people. (See the Resource Guide for details.)

We're a lucky generation of women who may not have it all, but we do have a lot: We can lead full and interesting lives with or without kids, and thanks to fertility drugs and treatments for PCOS, we have choices. But like it or not, PCOS does put the spotlight on fertility, and by doing so, it's instrumental in prompting you to make decisions about what your priorities and possibilities in life are. By focusing on what you want from life and how important motherhood may be, you can emerge with a stronger sense of identity. Seen in this light, the "baby or not" issue becomes an exciting voyage of self-discovery, helping you set the course for the rest of your life.

Area Two: Trying to Have a Baby

If you do decide to, or are currently trying to, have a baby, PCOS can add an extra dimension of worry and anxiety to the entire process, with the constant question *Will it happen?* going around inside your head. It can make sex and the rest of your relationship stressful; you can feel under pressure to do everything right with your diet, exercise, and lifestyle because you know it will be beneficial; and if you're not careful, every little thing you think you haven't done perfectly can make you feel like a failure—whether it's not exercising one night because you're tired, craving junk food, or that ultimate feeling of frustration when your period arrives once again, showing that you're still not pregnant.

For couples going through this process, it can be good to know that other people are, too. Joining a support group and meeting other couples experiencing similar challenges can be a huge relief.

> *"Getting together with couples who were going through what we were really helped us feel less isolated. It also let us see that there was a funny side to it, such as when I'd phone my husband in the middle of a meeting with his bank manager because I was at my peak fertility, and he had to make hasty excuses and rush off. Laughing about it broke the tension and helped us have better, less mechanical sex."* — Bryony, 34 years old

You can get information and support from organizations set up especially for couples having problems getting pregnant (see the Resource Guide). Or you may prefer to contact a relationship counselor or sex therapist, since having an objective third party can help you talk more openly.

If that all sounds too daunting or too public, there are many useful books for couples with relationship or sex problems, or for couples going through fertility treatment. You could simply schedule some time to sit down and talk about your problems together.

The main thing is not to get so obsessed with the fertility aspect of your life that everything else suffers. Follow the 80/20 rule when it comes to improving your lifestyle: Doing well 80 percent of the time is enough, as it gives you the room for treats and a night off. If you think about the fact that it takes average couples without PCOS around a year to conceive, you can take the pressure off yourself in terms of how fast you expect to succeed. And most of all, remember that more than 70 percent of women with PCOS do get pregnant naturally, so the odds are in your favor.

Area Three: The Highs and Lows of Fertility Treatment

If you decide that you do want kids and are considering or undertaking treatment for infertility, don't underestimate the emotional impact of this treatment. Finding out that you need medical help is a challenge, and one that will probably take you by surprise.

"When we got married, we expected to start a family within a year. I knew a couple who was going for IVF, but I never thought it would happen to us. It was a huge shock when I was diagnosed with PCOS. Equally shocking was the realization that once we began treatment, our problems weren't solved. I thought that medical science had an answer for everything, and I thought Clomid would do the trick, but it didn't. Then I assumed that IVF would make it happen, but that didn't work either. I'm about to begin my third cycle of IVF next month, and I'm beginning to realize that doctors still don't know that much about the seemingly simple task of getting pregnant." — Laura, 34 years old

"We were so anxious, unhappy, moody, and worried about money that after three cycles, we decided to take some time off and discuss if it was worth all the heartache. That really helped, because spending time together made us see that however much we wanted a baby, we still wanted to be with each other more." — Maria, 39 years old

"Coping with fertility treatment can be like coping with bereavement. Couples go through as many emotions—shock, anger, denial—every single month," says Anna McGrail, child-care expert and author of *Infertility: The Last Secret.* The constant failure as time goes by can strike deep at a woman's sense of self, and there may be days when all the joy seems to go out of life. You may even wonder whether you should continue treatment.

"The struggle takes over your life. I often stop and wonder how it might have been if I was normal and could have babies easily. Some days I wonder why I'm punishing myself over and over again when I may never conceive. I'm tired of living in a permanent state of crisis." — Mary

Acknowledge the Stress

Fertility treatment can take over your life, interfering with your relationships, your sex life, and your work. The entire invasive process can be exhausting and expensive. Many women say they find that their world shrinks. Timing is crucial if the drugs and treatments are to stand a chance of success, and all your attention needs to be focused on getting it right. According to Alice Domar, director of the Mind/Body Center for Women's Health at the Beth Israel Deaconess Medical Center in Boston, women trying to get pregnant can have stress levels (in terms of anxiety and depression) equivalent to women with cancer, HIV, and heart disease.

"Conception can become the main focus of your life, putting you on a roller-coaster ride that ends with dashed hopes once a month when your period arrives. Tracking ovulation can take all the fun and spontaneity out of sex, and marital disruption is common," says Joan Borysenko.

Many women are prepared to risk everything if there's even a tiny chance of becoming a mother: after all, there's always the hope that maybe the treatment will work next time. . . .

"We tried for two years before seeing a doctor. When I was diagnosed with PCOS, I freaked out because I've always wanted babies. What if I'd waited too long? We had test after test after test and five cycles of Clomid, but still no baby. Even more heartbreaking was that on one cycle I did get pregnant, but I miscarried at week ten. I really broke down then, and it took a lot of courage to start another cycle, this time on Pergonal. Thank

goodness I did, because that was the cycle I finally conceived my son." — Nicola, 35 years old

"When we decided to start a family, I knew that PCOS might cause problems, so I went to see my doctor right away. I was 36, and my physician warned me that there could be problems. After I don't know how many cycles of Clomid, I was told that I needed to see a specialist, but because of my age, the state health system couldn't treat me. Even if I'd been younger, I still would have had to spend years on the waiting list. Steven and I decided to take a risk and pay for private treatment, and we were very lucky: I got pregnant with twins. I know lots of people who have several courses of IVF and don't get pregnant, but it worked for us the first time. Life's wonderful now." — Laura, 37 years old

Agree on a Limit

Harder still is the constant waiting for appointments, tests, referrals, more tests, the results of tests, a medical procedure, the results of the procedure, funding decisions, treatment options, ovulation, more results, and still more tests. . . . You should be prepared to decide how far you're willing to go with your treatment. If you pay for it yourself rather than depending on insurance coverage, most clinics will recommend four treatments with IVF. If you want to keep going, a lot depends on how much your body and mind can endure, but it's important that you know when to stop trying—and that you remember you *do* have a choice. If you're in a relationship, communication with your partner is vital, because you both must agree on what the limit is. If you're single, you need to have an idea in your mind of how far you're willing to go.

Coping with the stress, anxiety, shock, and uncertainty of fertility treatment is exhausting and stressful. It can damage your self-esteem and your relationship. What makes it harder is the fact that many couples are reluctant to talk about their problems, preferring to keep things to themselves, but isolation at a time in your life when you feel most vulnerable is an added burden.

> *"I just can't talk to anyone about the way I feel. We keep it very quiet. If things go wrong, I don't think I could cope if people knew, but the trouble is that I feel as if I'm living a lie. People say how lucky we are to have our freedom and to take all those vacations. How can I tell them that what we really want is a child to share our 'wonderful' life with?"* — Lily, 36 years old

Staying Sane, Happy, and Positive Throughout the Fertility Journey

How do you manage the emotional roller coaster of any one of these PCOS fertility situations? How do you ensure that you don't feel isolated, guilty, or totally controlled by unpredictable emotions? This four-step action plan can help you weather the storm in a positive frame of mind.

Step One: Building Your Self-Esteem

Your sense of womanhood and femininity can take a beating when you have PCOS and its symptoms, such as excess hair, male-pattern baldness, weight gain that hides feminine curves, and no periods. How do you deal with these if you're finding it difficult to get pregnant, or if you're trying to get pregnant with that shadow hanging over you?

> *"I don't feel attractive anymore. Getting in the mood for sex is really difficult because all I see when I look in the mirror is this shapeless, plump woman with a light mustache and thinning hair. I can't understand what my husband sees in me. I don't have periods, and because of that I don't feel like a normal woman. I've always wanted a large family, and now I'm not sure I can*

even get pregnant. I feel like a failure. My body isn't working prop-erly, and I don't feel feminine." — Sophie, 34 years old

When your body doesn't do what it's expected to, you don't look the way you think you should, and you feel betrayed by your body, it's a huge blow to your self-esteem.

"Your level of self-esteem," says Boston psychotherapist and author of *Women & Self-Esteem*, Linda Tschirhart Sanford, "affects virtually everything we think, say and do. It affects how we see the world and our place in it. It affects how others treat us, the choices we make, our ability to give and receive love, and our ability to take action to change things that need to be changed. If a woman has an insufficient amount of self-esteem, she won't be able to act in her own best interests."

Low self-esteem can gradually destroy the quality of your life. You start to take less and less care of yourself. Your relationships, your sex life, and your work suffer. You sell yourself short by decid-ing that you aren't good enough before you start anything, which means that you don't put in the effort—and consequently, you end up fulfilling your idea that you aren't any good.

When you decide to go ahead with fertility treatment, a healthy sense of self-esteem is important. The process is a huge commitment, and you need to feel good about yourself to maximize your chances of success—remember how damaging emotional stress can be to your fertility. Accepting that you have self-esteem issues and tack-ling them now can help you avoid a downward spiral. It's been said many times before, but thinking positively and putting more emphasis on the good things in your life are great ways to build your self-esteem. No one says this is easy, but here are a few ideas to get you thinking along the right lines:

1. "You feel the way you think," says Dr. David Burns, a clini-cal psychiatrist at the Stanford University School of Medicine. "Negative feelings don't actually result from the bad things that hap-pen to you, but from the way you think about these events." If you think and talk negatively or always put yourself down, sooner or

later you'll end up believing those thoughts. A powerful self-esteem booster is to make an effort to **fill your thoughts and language with positive, liberating messages.** For example, avoid saying *I can't* or *I'm useless,* and substitute the statements *I'll try my best* or *I'm getting better.*

2. You'll turn problems into challenges and fear into excitement when you **accentuate the positive.** Avoid *should* and *ought,* replacing them with *could.* When something goes wrong, remember to put it into perspective. It's just one event—that doesn't mean you'll always get it wrong. Don't think *I've failed;* think *I'm learning new things all the time, and I'll know better next time.* Instead of *I've got PCOS, I'm never going to lose weight, and I may not be able to have babies;* try *PCOS is encouraging me to take better care of my health and appearance, and it's focusing my attention on how I can maximize my chances of having a healthy baby if and when the time is right.*

3. You're bound to feel better if you **bring fun and laughter into your life.** It's all too easy to get stuck in a complaining rut and focus on the serious side of life. Make room for some playtime, whether it's watching a funny movie, spending time with a friend who always lifts your spirits, or reading your favorite book. And smile more: Smiling can help you stop feeling bad about yourself and encourage others to communicate with you.

4. If others aren't valuing you, it's because you're letting them behave that way. Ask yourself why you're allowing it to happen, and then **teach other people how to treat you**—change the relationship by changing your behavior. Act assertively, and people who've been acting like you're a doormat will either modify their actions or leave your life.

An assertive woman knows what she wants, respects her own wishes, believes she can make things happen—and does, isn't afraid to say no or take a chance, accepts responsibility for her actions, expresses her true feeling, and respects and values the feelings of others. Above all, though, she values herself.

5. Another way to boost your self-esteem is to just **do something.** If you've been promising yourself that you'll learn a language, take a class, decorate your home, get a new wardrobe or a makeover, call your parents, clean the house, or take a vacation, then make sure you stop procrastinating and do it. Get rid of guilt and get started! You'll feel so much better, and this good feeling will encourage you to make even more positive changes in your life.

Try doing something creative such as painting a picture, writing a letter, or baking a cake. It's amazing how quickly your interest in life can be recaptured when you encourage yourself to use your creativity. And why not do something you've never tried before? Encourage your natural curiosity with a concert, an activity, a trip, or a class. When you do something for the first time, you'll experience a charge of energy and learn new things about yourself.

6. **Write an appreciation list.** If you're feeling blue, find things that you're grateful for, no matter how small. You may have to search hard, but it's worth the effort. The act of appreciation is the foundation of self-esteem.

7. If your friend or partner did something well, you'd want to reward them, so **be kind to yourself,** too. The next time you feel pleased because you've done a good job, honor yourself with a treat, a trip, a meal, or some leisure time. If you don't think you do anything well, then spend time focusing on your strengths. Make a list of all the things you know you're good at, from dealing with people to making a chocolate cake to being on time. You'll be surprised at the lift it gives you to concentrate on your positive strengths.

8. **Stop comparing yourself to other people.** Remember that you're unique. There never was and never will be another person on this planet like you, which makes you one of kind—special. Whenever you feel the urge to fit in, just accept your differences and make the most of them. They're what make you a unique and original person with your own place in the world.

9. Don't wait until you lose weight, have a partner, get pregnant, or get a promotion to love yourself. **Start loving yourself today,** and don't put off life. Tell yourself over and over again that you're lovable for who you are, not for what you look like or what you do. At first, it may seem weird and unbelievable, but do it often enough, and it will start to become a habit. And when things become habits, they become part of who you are. Self-confidence is our birthright: Just look at any newborn, and you can see that it wants and expects love. Lack of self-confidence is something that's happened to you along the path of life and turned into a bad habit, perhaps because of negative messages from others. Break that pattern and replace it with self-confidence. After all, it's who you were meant to be.

10. When you feel really low, try this wonderful technique to lift yourself out of negativity. Imagine that you've stepped out of your body and are standing next to yourself. **Become your own best friend.** Now, what would you say to yourself that's comforting and helpful? How can you encourage this person to feel more confident about herself? What would you say to your best friend? Perhaps you'd put your arm around her, tell her that she's doing really well, and that you appreciate all the good things about her. Talk to yourself the way you would to your best friend.

Body Image

Working through the PCOS issues surrounding your body image is an important part of building your self-esteem and nourishing your sex life. Body image and self-esteem are intimately linked. The danger lies in letting your negative attitudes toward your body make you feel like a failure in all aspects of your life.

The great majority of women worry about the way they look. A 2003 survey of 45,000 women carried out by the Women's Channel of AOL found that only 4 percent of women were happy with their looks, and around two-thirds feel uncomfortable with the way they look. Worrying about their figure was an everyday occurrence for

41 percent of women, with 26 percent of that number saying it bothered them most when clothes shopping.

Most of us aren't entirely happy with our physical selves, from ears that we think stick out to a stomach that sags. Other people may see us far less critically, and this is the difference between our bodies and our body image. "Restoring and maintaining a positive body image when you have PCOS, especially when you are trying for a baby, can be extremely hard. And putting on weight, finding excess facial hair, losing hair from your head, dull skin, acne, and worrying about fertility due to absent or irregular periods can all have a hugely damaging effect on your body image," says Dr. Helen Mason of St. George's Hospital Medical School, London.

There are two important steps you need to take if you want to feel less negative about your body: (1) Learning to be happy with the body you have, and (2) forgiving yourself for not looking the way you think you ought to look. These are very difficult processes to achieve, but they're by no means impossible.

A positive body image makes any woman look attractive, regardless of how much she weighs or what she looks like. It's confidence that makes someone look sexy, not a tiny waist and a big bust, and by working on your self-esteem and body image, you can build your confidence.

So stop trying to change your appearance, and start transforming the way you feel about how you look. Taking the following small steps to a more positive body image can slowly help you feel happier about yourself. (*Note:* If your body-image problems are leading you to develop an unhealthy relationship with food, contact the eating-disorders support groups listed in the Resource Guide for help, support, advice, and information.)

1. It goes without saying that the first step has to be doing all you can to **try to ease your PCOS symptoms.** This will involve visiting your doctor and following the healthful diet, exercise, and lifestyle advice in our fertility-boosting plan. Exercise is particularly helpful, and the buzz you get from having spent time on yourself will make you look and feel good.

2. **Talk about it.** Try discussing why you feel so uncomfortable about your body with people you trust, such as family, friends, or other women with PCOS. Is there something in particular that makes you feel self-conscious, or do you only feel that way in certain circumstances? Why do you think your life will be better when you lose weight, have clear skin, or have shiny, healthy hair? Read some celebrity magazines, and you'll find lots of stories about unhappy thin women with perfect skin and hair. You don't have to look a certain way in order to feel healthy, happy, and energized.

3. Taking some time to think about how you want to look will help you face the world with more confidence, so **give yourself a makeover.** It could involve a new haircut, wardrobe, or shade of lipstick. Perhaps you'd like to seek the advice of a fashion expert to find out what styles flatter you. Steer clear of darker colors if you're feeling sad, and wear brighter, more cheerful ones instead. Unusual accessories can focus other people's attention away from any problems you think you have with your body. And don't underestimate the importance of a bra that fits properly: It can do wonders for your figure.

4. Do yourself a favor and **throw out your old clothes.** Do you have things that you never wear or that you used to love but are too small now? Get rid of them. They're a constant reminder that you haven't lost weight, and living in the past isn't good for your self-esteem and body image. Give them to someone who can enjoy them.

5. **Stand tall** and think about your posture. You'll feel more streamlined and more confident about your body if you stand, walk, and sit properly. Try reminding yourself to sit properly at your desk on the hour every hour, and you'll be surprised how quickly you develop better habits. Or try a course in Alexander technique to realign your posture permanently.

6. It's not how you look but how you feel about the way you look that matters. **Think positively** about your body. If you had a friend who kept saying you were fat and ugly, she wouldn't stay your

friend for long, so don't tolerate that kind of treatment from your-self either. If you find this difficult, take a good look at yourself in the mirror. At first you'll see all the parts you don't like, but in time you'll also notice what you do find attractive: an inviting twinkle in your eyes, the seductive curve of your shoulders, a womanly tummy. Start respecting your body. (Also, review our natural tips for boosting libido in Chapter 2.)

Step Two: Strengthening Your Relationship with Your Partner

Your relationship with your partner can also come under intense strain during the PCOS fertility roller-coaster ride. Many women with this condition talk about the huge burden it places on a rela-tionship if there's difficulty conceiving or they end up not having children. Other women say how hard it is to get in the mood for sex when they've gained weight or when acne, facial hair, and absent periods make them feel less feminine. Fertility drugs can also take their toll, and having sex because your doctor says you have to can dampen any couple's enthusiasm.

If you feel that PCOS, anxiety about your fertility, and/or the treat-ments for it are negatively affecting your sex life, then it's important to get to the root of the problem. First, your sex life could simply be affected by a busy schedule, stress at work, or financial worries. Solv-ing these problems can give your relationship a new lease on life.

Take Time to Talk

It could just be that you've stopped talking to each other about how you feel. "With increasing honesty as you voice your feelings," says relationship expert and author Steve Biddulph, "a couple can begin to understand and clear up obstacles to closeness one by one. Love grows through the vulnerability you show, as well as the strength of feelings you admit to." Try making a pact for a week that as soon as you see each other at the end of the day, no matter how late it is, you'll talk for ten minutes about the kind of day you had, and then for ten minutes about how the day and/or how the fertility treatment affected you emotionally. This way, you give each other support and build up intimacy that can otherwise get lost.

Talking about Sex

It can be embarrassing to talk about sex, especially if it hasn't been occurring or you aren't enjoying it, so how can you initiate a conversation? It helps to make the issue a shared one by asking your partner what he thinks or how he feels about your sex life. Admit that you find it embarrassing, but let him know that the relationship means a lot to you and you want to start communicating. And once the issue is out in the open, don't suddenly feel that you must have intensely passionate sex all the time. It's important that you don't feel under pressure to perform just because you've brought up the subject.

Put the emphasis on romance, not sex. Spending more time together as a couple, whether it's during a jog in the morning, a picnic in the park, a candlelit bath, or a special evening meal, can help bring you closer so that you start seeing yourselves as lovers again. Make an effort to have fun. Remember, sex is supposed to be enjoyable, not a battleground. Try things together that you haven't done before, share jokes, or do something a little crazy, such as dancing in the rain. It doesn't matter what you do as long as it's harmless and makes you both laugh.

Perhaps your relationship and your sex life have gotten into a rut because they've started to seem functional, rather than fun and spontaneous expressions of your love and desire for each other as a couple.

"I don't think of pleasure anymore when I'm having sex. I think about the drugs I'm taking, the timing, my next doctor's appointment, and how much I want to have a baby. My husband feels under pressure, and that doesn't help either of us—he once

said that he feels like a sperm bank and nothing more." — Pat,
40 years old

Try breaking out of this perspective by focusing on the pleasure and bonding experience for you as a couple. Try adding some
variety into your daily and nightly routines: Get up at different
times, eat new kinds of food, and experiment with new sexual
positions and fresh places.

Don't wait until you feel good about yourself to be more dar-
ing—try it now. Doing new things and taking risks in and out of bed
can make you feel more alive and more attractive.

Physical symptoms of PCOS can also take their toll on your
desire to be intimate. If you don't see yourself as a sexual being anymore, rediscover your passionate side by spending time on yourself.
Some women find masturbation helpful when they aren't having
a particularly close experience in their relationship.

If you feel self-conscious about your weight, acne, or body hair,
address those issues directly by buying some provocative underwear,
getting some new perfume, or having a facial or a bikini wax.

Plan for Romance

It may help to plan romance a little more. Schedule a time when
you and your partner know that you'll be alone together. This doesn't
always mean you'll have sex; it means that you'll share intimate
moments together. You might end up taking a walk or cuddling in
front of the TV. In that special time, many things may spontaneously
happen, and one of them might be sex.

Perhaps by midweek, you and your partner can agree that on a
Saturday you'll spend a romantic evening together. By planning,
you can set aside time on that day to concentrate on feeling your best.
You could try something fairly extreme, like getting a new hairstyle
at your salon, or something simple like taking a nice nap so you don't
feel tired in the evening. You want to look forward to this, not feel
as if it's hard work.

Show Some Affection

If you aren't in the mood because you feel anxious, worried, or tired, why not initiate intimacy instead of withdrawing from it? Don't shut out your partner; hold hands or ask for a hug instead. Make an effort to show physical affection, and then receive it when it's offered. You'll be surprised how supported, accepted, and lovable it makes you feel.

Above all, if you're finding that sex is a problem, *don't ignore it.* It's an important part of a committed relationship, so use books, therapy, videos, or whatever works best for you—any good relationship is worth the work. (Also see our advice on pages 65–75 in Chapter 2.)

Remember, This Isn't Your Fault!

If PCOS is the reason you aren't getting pregnant, it can be hard for you not to blame yourself or feel betrayed by your body. You may also feel anxious that your partner will somehow feel let down.

"I feel so guilty because I've got it all—a lovely husband, a great job, and a good life—but I can't do the one thing that would make our lives perfect: get pregnant. Simon reassures me that he loves me whether or not we have kids, but a part of me feels that I've let him down because he loves children, and he'd be a fantastic dad. If we stay childless, will he turn against me one day? I'm scared of that, and I sometimes think that it would be better for him if he was with someone who could give him a family." — Chloe, 32 years old

This may sound harsh, but filling a hole in your relationship or making your partner happy aren't good reasons to have children. It's understandable if your partner feels let down, disappointed, or angry, but if your relationship is strong enough, you'll work through it. If you can't, then you should ask yourself if your relationship was that strong in the first place.

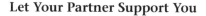

Let Your Partner Support You

A relationship is about loving someone for who they are, including their imperfections. Turn the tables: If your partner had a low sperm count, would you reject him? No, of course you wouldn't, because you love him. So expect him to show the same kind of devotion to you, and don't retreat into yourself or push him away.

PCOS isn't something you should fight on your own. Let your partner help so that you can make decisions about the situation together. This will show you whether you really have the right support from him, and it's better to discover this now than when you're six months pregnant.

Talking about your relationship and sex life can help you understand how your partner feels about PCOS, and how it and the fertility treatments are affecting things. Without realizing it, you may be unconsciously pushing him away. You might be convinced that he's disappointed in you because you aren't fertile, or isn't attracted to you because of PCOS symptoms such as weight gain and acne, only to find that he wants to help you and get close to you again but doesn't know how to go about it.

Try not to withdraw from your partner at this crucial time, even if you're afraid that he might say things you don't want to hear. Include him in the process at all times because this concerns both of you, and you need to understand how your partner feels: He's trying to have a baby, too, and wants to help you stop feeling terrible about yourself because it isn't happening.

Initiating discussions and exploring your feelings together (about why you can't get pregnant or why you're spending money on fertility treatments, for example) can help you discover how much PCOS affects your shared life. It can also help you find out whether or not your relationship is really ready for a child.

Above all, stop blaming yourself if PCOS is making it hard for you to get pregnant. Sure, there are things you can do to ease your symptoms (such as healthful eating and regular exercise), but at the end of the day, it remains a condition that you're susceptible to for some reason. "We don't know enough about PCOS yet to have all the answers," says Adam Balen, "but we do know for sure that it isn't your fault if you have it."

Step Three: Ease Emotional Stress

Just thinking about having a baby can be stressful. Even while you're using ovulation-predictor kits, you may be worrying about whether you'll be able to handle the 24-hour responsibility of a baby and, as we saw above, trying to make this decision can be one of the first major challenges.

"The stressful nature of trying for a baby with or without fertility treatment is now recognized by experts the world over," says Harvard infertility specialist Alice Domar. Letting yourself cry can help, as can talking to your partner or other women with PCOS, but learning how to manage your feelings so that you don't have as many bad days is even better.

Incorporating the following stress-management habits into your life can help you avoid much of the tension associated with baby making. If you want to protect your relationship and the health and well-being of yourself and your partner, as well as increase your chances of getting pregnant (remember, stress has a negative effect on fertility), we suggest the following guidelines:

1. **Continue the healthful eating and exercise plan** outlined in Chapter 2 because physical well-being is an important part of controlling stress. Lack of exercise can also make you feel restless and anxious, so get active. Simply walking is a great stress reliever, so add it to your routine.

2. **Nurture yourself** with relaxation techniques such as deep breathing from the abdomen (not the chest), meditation, prayer, guided imagery, or yoga; or simply zone out and daydream every so often. Allow your mind to wander for five minutes every time you feel tense. Maybe use a favorite picture or holiday memory to help

you daydream, or discover places that you find relaxing and spend some time there as often as possible, even if it's only ten minutes in the park at lunchtime.

3. **Be good to yourself.** In scientific studies, feeling pleasure (particularly when it involves our senses), has been found to enhance not only our sense of well-being, but our health, too. For example, gazing at an attractive aquarium of tropical fish relaxes us, as well as lowers our blood pressure. Music, pleasant aromas, and the tastes of certain foods have also been used successfully to calm people and reduce pain, depression, and stress.

Think hard about what would give you pleasure. It doesn't have to be anything expensive—you can treat yourself to a bunch of flowers, a manicure, and a new mystery novel. Take a long bath, preferably with a wonderful oil or aromatherapy scent (classic essential oils to reduce stress include geranium, lavender, neroli, and Roman chamomile). Spend some time by yourself or get together with women whose lives aren't centered around children. You can also join a book club, window shop, go camping with your partner, watch more movies, or spend a weekend in the country and forget what time it is. Whatever you enjoy, think of it as a doctor's prescription for your health, and do it regularly.

4. **Practice mindfulness,** the technique of living in the here-and-now and enjoying the present moment. One of the peculiar effects of infertility is that it tends to be so totally absorbing. You're concentrating on the next step in your treatment, what your ovulation-predictor kit will reveal, whether you had enough sex when you ovulated, and so on. Soon, there's no room in your mind for what's actually going on around you. By being mindful and focusing on every aspect of what you're doing—whether eating lunch, walking down the street, or completing another task—you're both relaxing and nurturing yourself. Your feelings of being stressed out vanish as you focus on finding pleasure in the present moment.

The activity you choose doesn't matter—it can be as simple as peeling an orange. What's important is your awareness as you go about it. Take your time: Peel the fruit slowly, notice its fragrance and color, and pay attention to how it tastes. Remember that the purpose of mindfulness is the deliberate cultivation of your awareness of the here-and-now. You can take a walk, eat a meal, or make love mindfully. The key is to slow down and engage all your senses in what you're doing. Don't worry if your mind wanders. This is entirely normal, so learn to watch each thought as it comes and goes, not fighting it, but just gently turning your attention back to the task in hand.

5. **Express your emotions.** Not surprisingly, anger is one of the strongest feelings women with PCOS often have. You may feel angry at your body for betraying you, other people for not understanding, the constant waiting, and women who do have kids because it seems so unfair. Expressing your emotions in a journal—even for just ten minutes a day—can help you come to terms with much of the negative burden you may not even realize you're carrying. Don't limit yourself to angry feelings, but instead, use your journal to write down all your emotions: grief, fear, hope, disgust, and self-discovery. You might gain fresh insights into your situation.

6. **Find or form a support group** of women with PCOS who are experiencing infertility, whether in your local area or through e-mail or the Internet. (PCOS support groups are also discussed in the next section of this chapter and in the Resource Guide.) If infertility is causing severe anxiety, ask your doctor for help or search for professional counseling. And if it's creating severe problems in your relationship, consider couples counseling with a therapist who specializes in treating those suffering from infertility. If your partner won't join you, go alone.

Step Four: Finding Support

If you're trying to have a baby, you'll obviously rely on your partner as a huge source of support and backup. He will know very well what you've gone through in trying to deal with PCOS-related symptoms, and the best way to make sure you both aren't overwhelmed is to be up front about your feelings and share what you're experiencing.

In addition to your partner, it's also important to gather a network of support. If you don't have a partner, such a group is absolutely crucial for helping you cope with the emotional side of PCOS and fertility treatment. Your doctor and fertility specialist are there for you to share medical issues with. Partners, family members, and friends can learn more about PCOS, attend support-group meetings or doctors' appointments with you, and ask what else they can do for you: Perhaps your mom knows the perfect way to cheer you up, your sister can help you stick to a healthful diet, and close friends can motivate you to keep fit. Tell them why exercise is important for your health and well-being, educate them about your condition, and they'll be there for you.

Difficulties with Family

Support from the people who care about you is simply the best, but unfortunately, it may not always come automatically, especially if they don't know anything about PCOS, have kids already, have never worried about getting pregnant, or happen to live far away. It will also be difficult for them if you're not comfortable sharing your concerns.

Dealing with family can be challenging if you're expected to attend celebrations where children are present, and there will be times when you just can't deal with it.

"Christmas has always been hard for Simon and me, and two years ago, we both came back home in tears. I took and failed a pregnancy test on Christmas Eve, and then had to join in the extended-family celebrations. We felt envious of everyone's joy and seeing the children open their presents. In the New Year, I told my mom why I wasn't getting pregnant, but I wish I hadn't. She

just keeps giving me pearls of wisdom that makes things worse, like 'You've got plenty of time' or 'Relax and it will happen.' She just doesn't understand." — Rachel, 44 years old

Difficulties with Friends

Things can be just as upsetting with your friends. "Every one," says Sally, "and I mean *every one* of my friends has children now." If this is the case, you could feel as if you've become the odd one out. It's a lonely feeling, and it's happening just when you really need to talk to someone. As months pass and you still haven't conceived, you may be surprised by how angry and jealous you feel when you see someone who's pregnant or has a baby, or just hearing about them. And because you're of childbearing age, you'll probably be surrounded by evidence of others' fertility.

It's not uncommon for women with PCOS fertility problems to withdraw from their social lives, even to the point that they cease to talk on the phone with anyone who has a child. As a result, they feel more isolated and different than ever from people who were once a part of their support system.

"I've found it so difficult to stay in touch with and share the lives of several of my once-good friends. Every time I see their kids, I feel annoyed and jealous, and for some reason, they can't seem to talk about anything else because their whole lives revolve around their families now.

"Getting them to find a babysitter for a girls' night out is such hard work that it makes me feel like I'm imposing. And anyway, I know that at some point they'll want to talk about how I'm doing in my attempts to get pregnant. They'll try to be supportive, when really I just want them to take my mind off it for once." — Sue, 36 years old

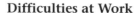
Difficulties at Work

It can also be hard to know whether to tell co-workers or not. If you do, they may jump to the wrong conclusions and put your career on hold, thinking that you may get pregnant at any moment, not to mention continually asking the inevitable "Are you pregnant yet?" questions. But if you don't let them know, what are you going to say when you need to take time off for tests and appointments? If you don't say anything, you could create even more stress as you invent reasons for your absences.

What Can You Do?

How do you deal with your own expectations and those of others when you're riding the PCOS fertility roller coaster?

"You need to find the people you can trust whom you want to share your emotions, feelings, and stresses with," says Dominique, who's 35 years old and currently pregnant with her first child. *"When we first decided to try to have a baby, I realized that I wanted to tell my closest friend about my fears because of PCOS, but that I didn't want to tell anyone else so that I could just go out and feel 'normal' when I was with them.*

"But after more than a year of trying with no success, I widened my circle of confidantes to include a couple more friends and a colleague at work who'd told me that she was finding it difficult to get pregnant, too. That way, it wasn't always just my husband I was letting off steam with, and I felt much less stress."

"I'd say to anyone coping with the PCOS fertility question that you'll find your own time to tell people," says Kerri, age 42, who now has two children. *"But swallowing your pride and*

asking for support is often the best thing you can do. I found it hard because I first had to explain what PCOS was to several of my friends and my three sisters. But once I had, they were so good—and in fact, it turned out that the sister I'd never been really close to also had PCOS, but hadn't ever told me. So we ended up supporting each other in a really unexpected way."

Talking to loved ones, friends, and colleagues about the frustrations you have with PCOS and your fertility treatments can really help. People aren't mind readers—unless you let them know what's going on, they can't support you. Never underestimate how much those around you want to listen, understand, and be there for you, or how much you'll need them.

So help yourself and your partner through the rough times by gathering together your own support network, whether it's made up of friends or family members. If you can't do this or—worse still—have begun to stay away from family and friends, have no one to talk with about your feelings, or feel abnormal because you don't have a child and can't discuss it with your partner, it's time to seek outside help.

PCOS Support Groups

Support can come ready-made in the form of a PCOS support group (see the Resource Guide) where contacts, group meetings, advice, Websites, chat rooms, and information for women trying to conceive will be available.

"The emotional support from other women who have PCOS and fertility issues is invaluable. Peer support offers the ability to talk freely about the issues you've been dealing with. It can be especially wonderful to talk with others who have firsthand knowledge of what you're going through." — Kristin, 33 years old

Hospital Support Groups

Also check your local hospital for fertility-support groups. Many hospitals have them, and although you may not find as many people with your condition as you would in a PCOS-specific group, you'll meet couples and other women who are also struggling to have children.

Whatever your personal situation, support groups are out there. Even if you feel that you want to cope with PCOS and/or fertility treatment alone, the sense of security you can get from knowing that there are others you can turn to in times of disappointment, uncertainty, and crisis is a huge comfort.

Stop Explaining

The important thing is to get beyond feeling that you need to explain yourself to anyone else, and spend some time managing your condition and de-stressing instead. Of course, it's your choice how up front you are with others, but remember that the more people who know about PCOS and how it impacts your fertility, the less explaining you'll need to do . . . and that also means less explaining for the millions of other women with PCOS concerned about their fertility.

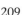

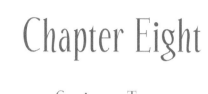

Chapter Eight

Coming to Terms
with Loss and Moving Forward

If you reach the point where you decide that having children isn't going to happen for you, it can be a shock. But it's a sad fact that while many women with PCOS are eventually able to have children, many others experience miscarriage along the way, and some finally have to cope with their inability to have children at all.

You'll need lots of space, time, and support to accept that you need to move to a different path and find a new set of values and coping skills. It may be even harder to accept that one day these values will feel fulfilling—although couples who've been through the transition say that it does happen, albeit slowly.

> "At the time, it seemed like our world had come to an end. We were numb with shock and grief, but the things we went through have made us stronger—both as individuals and as a couple—and without realizing it, we channeled our creativity into other areas of our life: our jobs, friends, and family. We've survived, and our lives didn't stand still—even though we couldn't see that at the time." — Steve and Mandy

You're going to feel an entire range of intense emotions. In addition to a huge sense of loss and pain, you may feel as if you've failed. You may grieve that your genes won't continue on or that your creativity—so deeply connected to your sexuality—seems to be blocked.

You may feel as if you've lost your female identity, that your inability to experience motherhood isolates you from other women, a sense of guilt about previous lifestyle choices to abort or postpone a baby, or anger because you didn't seek help for PCOS earlier.

"Every time I see a mother, I feel as if I've failed in some way. I've lost my spark, my zest for life. I hope, I pray, I hope, I curse, I hope, and I wish. Some days, I feel that I don't want to go on if I can't have a baby." — Sarah, 42 years old

"It makes me so angry. Even people who've struggled to have kids complain about them. How easily they forget their tremendous luck—and those who became parents easily have no idea how lucky they are either!" — Marion, 37 years old

"I feel such pain that I may never have a baby grow inside me. I know I have lots of good things in my life, but there's something missing. Why do I long to be a mother? I don't know. All I know is that the future without children looks empty." — Louise, 30 years old

"I know lots of women put off having babies because the timing isn't right. But if you've got PCOS, you have to be aware that the longer you wait, the more you reduce your chances compared to other women. That's what happened to me. I thought I could wait until my late 30s, but I ended up losing baby after baby, and spending time and money I didn't have on fertility treatment. Nothing worked, and the whole ordeal nearly destroyed me. I can't describe the anguish I felt after each miscarriage—that huge sense of sadness, loss, and failure will never leave me. The day I

finally decided to stop putting myself through this monthly torment was a relief, but it was also the bleakest, blackest day of my life."
— Susie

Give Yourself Permission to Feel

How on earth do you come to terms with this maelstrom of feelings and get to a stage where you can move on with your life when you still see babies, pregnant women, and children laughing everywhere you go? All your friends have kids, and they belong to a secret world organized around child care. They look exhausted and stressed, but you envy their busy child-filled lives and ache with sadness at the empty space in your own.

First, you need to let yourself understand that you're not crazy or weak to be feeling like an emotional wreck. The stress on both you and your partner can be overwhelming, and experts acknowledge that the hugely traumatic experience of infertility can make or break a couple because it damages self-esteem, triggers many complex emotions, and isolates you from the majority of other people. "In a world that values parenthood," says American fertility expert Robert Franklin, "infertile couples feel alone and different; they're often the only couple at the picnic or family reunion without children. Eventually they begin to feel as if they don't belong to this parent-oriented society—they feel abandoned and isolated."

Moving on with Your Life

Before you can move forward, you must say good-bye to your past. You can't have a baby, and right now, you may find it impossible to gather anything positive from what seems such a black and bitter experience, but if you can look your loss straight in the eye, you'll uncover a courage within. Saying farewell isn't easy, but grief closes the door behind you so that you can enter a new phase of life, with all the opportunities and possibilities it has to offer. The following practical steps are suggestions to help you get through the process of grieving and come to terms with your new life.

Learn New Coping Skills

Women struggling with infertility go through a roller coaster of emotions, but one of their biggest concerns is loss of control over their bodies and lives. "There is not a single person going through infertility who feels in control," says London-based infertility psychologist Sonia Heiger.

In addition, infertility can also throw your value system into chaos. Most of us are brought up to believe that through hard work, we can achieve pretty much anything, that there's justice in the world, and that if we do the right thing, life will treat us well in return. But as we've seen, infertility turns all this upside down. Most childless couples have worked hard to conceive and have lived decent lives, but justice still doesn't prevail.

The values that may have been governing your life until now might not be helping you deal with the experience of infertility, so in order to regain a sense of control over your life, you need to reexamine your standards, which can open up your mind to learning new coping skills.

Let Go of the Past

Guilt and pain from the past can reappear and drive the agony of infertility even deeper. A previous abortion, for example, can be one of the most painful memories to face, and it's difficult to not see your current infertility as a punishment. If this is the case, you need to reconsider the circumstances surrounding the abortion and understand that it was a loss and must be grieved in order to heal the pain and move forward.

Stop Judging Yourself by Your Fertility

"I've got this amazing career, but at times, I feel like I haven't really succeeded as a woman. It's crazy and un-PC, but without a child, I feel like I haven't achieved that much." — Mary

When you can't have a baby, it's because your reproductive process is breaking down, not because you or your partner are failures. It isn't easy, but you need to develop an accurate sense of self and understand that you're far more than just the ability to conceive. Try not to think that because this isn't working, nothing is. Having children is important, but if you're going to survive this, you must put it into perspective.

"Try to keep the focus narrow by reminding yourself that only a part of your body is infertile, not your entire being," says Harriette Rovner Ferguson, a New York psychotherapist specializing in infertility.

Even today, despite all the exciting options open to us women and all that we achieve, if we can't get pregnant, we may still think of ourselves as "less than" we should be. We still place a high premium on the role of mother, and not having children if we've been conditioned to think that it was our purpose in life can be a crushing blow to our self-worth. (If this is how you feel, see our advice in Chapter 7 on building self-esteem.)

Manage Stress Positively

You need to learn to manage the stress of infertility in a positive way. Healthful eating and regular exercise are great ways to reduce stress, as are talking with close friends and family and getting involved with infertility support groups. Staying positively focused and reminding yourself that it's the treatment that's failing—not you—will help you reframe the experience in a more positive light. If you have difficulty doing this, a professional counselor or therapist can help you change negative thinking about yourself and your life.

Coping with loss means that you give yourself permission to be angry and to cry. Anger is an important part of grieving, and you need to express it in order to release stress, but it's important to realize that your anger is directed at the problem and not at others—that is, not at your younger sister who has just gotten pregnant, your boss who has five kids, or the social worker who visits your home to see if it's suitable for adoption when you know that most people don't have to go through this.

Crying is important because grief is the body's natural healer for emotional loss. At times it may seem too painful, but the only way to heal is to let yourself feel the sorrow without guilt. If you refuse to face your grief, you'll never heal, and you may get stuck in that phase. (See the description of the Five Stages of Grief later in this chapter.)

Take Care of Your Partner, Too

Sharing your grief with someone you care about, preferably your partner, is the key to releasing bottled-up tension. When the two of you share your grief, you can grow closer, since communicating your vulnerability is the foundation of intimacy.

This doesn't mean that the hurt disappears; instead, the bond of understanding and affection grows. Problems tend to occur when one partner feels isolated from the other, and couples need to understand that infertility is "our" problem, not "my" problem.

"Although many marriages are strengthened during an infertility workup, the divorce rate is high among infertile couples, especially those who are unable to share their feelings," says Dr. Franklin, professor of gynecology at Baylor College of Medicine in Houston, Texas. So it's important to reach out to your partner and protect your relationship, since he's likely to being feeling as vulnerable and hurt as you are right now. Infertility doesn't have to do permanent damage to your union. The crisis can be a learning opportunity, a chance to discover more about your partner's coping style, as well as how to take better care of each other.

Accept That Men Cope Differently

Men are often more oriented toward solving problems, while women tend to vent their feelings, so expecting your partner to mirror your coping skills can be disappointing.

"I just wanted someone to hold me, listen, and say, 'Yes, it must be awful. You must feel terrible, and I sympathize,' but my partner didn't want to hold on to that sense of grief—or 'wallow in it,' as he put it. He'd say, 'Okay, if we can do this, do that, and try again, then we can have a baby next time.' He meant well in trying to be positive, but at the time, I just needed someone to acknowledge the depths of my hurt." — Emma, 33 years old

You may not get all that you need from your partner, so it might be helpful to supplement his support with what you receive from your friends and family.

Hone Your Communication Skills

In order to cope with infertility, you need good communication skills: Let your partner and the people close to you know how you want to be treated. Infertile women often say *what* the problem is, but they don't always let their listeners know *how* they feel or what they *need*. For example, compare, "I had a pregnancy test, and it was negative," with "I had a pregnancy test today, and it was negative. I feel miserable and hopeless and need to be held." The latter is more likely to be understood because the entire message is communicated, whereas the former leaves the listener uncertain about how to help.

Join a Support Group

Wherever you are in your fertility treatment—waiting for results, grieving, deciding to withdraw, or considering adoption—it's worth thinking about the various infertility support groups that exist both locally and nationally. Not only can they give you advice and information, but they can also put you in touch with other people going through the same thing, and they have numerous hotlines for particular issues and experiences.

You may find that you get all you need from a PCOS support group, or you might discover that general infertility organizations address more of your needs. Most (but not all) clinics also have patient support groups that can provide information, leaflets, addresses, and activities.

You may find the idea of joining a group scary or depressing since doing so acknowledges that you have a problem, but you don't have to go to meetings—you can pledge your support by staying in touch via reassuring and comforting newsletters or by visiting infertility-support Websites and chat rooms (see the Resource Guide for details).

The Five Stages of Grief

Since confronting grief can be intensely painful and overwhelming, we often try to protect ourselves by avoiding it, but this normal healing process has to be experienced in order for us to move forward. The last thing you may want to do is face it, but grief is the only way our bodies know how to heal the pain.

"Regardless of whether the grief is real (in response to an actual loss) or anticipated (when a treatment cycle fails), it must be experienced," says Dr. Franklin. "It is by experiencing our feelings through grief that we help them go away. If we fail to do this they linger, causing us suffering."

Research has shown that infertile couples need to allow themselves to grieve and to express their anger and anguish. Without such expression, the feelings remain unresolved, so it should help that the five stages outlined in the model below have now been applied to infertility counseling. We all go through this in different ways, but regardless of our personal style, there are predictable stages for everyone—although they don't always appear in the same order. If you're coping with the trauma of infertility, these changing emotions are entirely normal and natural.

Stage One: Shock and Denial

The first stage of grief is shock and/or denial. Even if you know that you have PCOS and that it can affect your fertility, you may still be stunned to discover that you have this problem. Once you can accept that the challenge exists, the diagnosis isn't so painful to hear, and you can begin to talk about it. Seek advice, help, and support, and move out of this stage.

Stage Two: Anger

Not being able to have children when you want to seems cruelly unfair. It's as if Nature has cheated you of your birthright, and you may well find yourself experiencing the *Why me?* syndrome: "When so many women can—and often shouldn't—have a baby, why can't I get pregnant?" This anger may increase to rage when you do everything humanly possible, but still don't get pregnant. Sometimes that anger may get directed away from yourself into *Why you?* and anyone who reminds you of your infertility will become the target of your anger: your partner, your sister with her beautiful new baby, your doctor, or pregnant women in world at large.

But the most harmful anger by far is the one that's directed against yourself. You may get so upset with yourself that your self-esteem falters, leaving only an overwhelming sense of failure.

Stage Three: Bargaining

Feeling desperate, you may start to bargain with God or a higher power in order to gain a feeling of control. You may actually believe that if you're a better person or do this or that good deed, then you'll become pregnant. Sadly, when the good deed doesn't translate into pregnancy, this can make you feel even more out of control, exhausted, and abandoned—as if you did your part, but the universe didn't respond.

Stage Four: Feeling Hopeless and Helpless

With every miscarriage or failed treatment, you may begin to feel more and more hopeless and helpless. This is the most vulnerable stage, when you could sink into a depression where there's no hope and no positive options. Many couples refer to this as the *black-hole stage.* You may experience it month after month when your hopes are dashed by a negative pregnancy test, or you may find yourself there when you finally decide to call it a day and stop treatment.

If this happens, the danger is that you'll lose your resilience and the ability to build up hope again, and you'll lack the mental energy to pull yourself through it. Professional help may be needed to help you learn more effective coping strategies.

Stage Five: Acceptance

The final stage involves accepting that there's a problem and that you may never be able to have a child of your own; you admit that you have a problem and that it hurts—it hurts a lot. Acceptance doesn't mean that your grieving is over, but that it's managed in a way that's healthy for you and your partner. Yes, you want a baby, but you accept that you can't have one and that it isn't your fault. The pain of this loss is a part of your life, but it doesn't control you because you find ways to cope with it. You may be able to do this alone, with family and friends, or with the support of a counselor or therapist.

Infertility Counseling

Counseling isn't the same as psychotherapy and psychoanalysis, which assume that deep disturbances that have their roots in childhood. This treatment starts from the idea of addressing the current issues in your life and exploring painful feelings associated with them. Infertility is a life crisis, and your health-care providers simply won't have the time to help you and your partner take stock of all the news that hits you.

Counseling provides a quiet space for the two of you to mull over your feelings and get the support and information you need. We'd urge any couple going through fertility treatment to include this—as a couple—in their treatment plan. Seeing a counselor doesn't mean that there's anything wrong with you, just that infertility is causing a range of turbulent emotions and you may need to talk about them with someone.

Professional counselors are an important part of any fertility clinic. They're medically informed and can help you make decisions about your treatment and cope with the consequences. We advise you to ask right at the beginning of your relationship with a clinic what their counseling service consists of, and if it's an added cost, how much it will be. If it's not included, you may prefer to see your GP and find out if his or her practice has an in-house counselor you could see, or you can find someone on your own.

There may be reasons that you don't want to go to counseling. For example, you might have your own way of coping that includes friends and family members who can give you all the support you need. That's fine, but we do recommend that you check out your clinic's counselor to see whether or not you might still benefit from the service.

Coping with Miscarriage

Miscarriage is far more common than you may realize, regardless of whether you have PCOS. An estimated 1 out of 4 women experience it, and 1 out of 300 have lost three or four pregnancies. But if you experience a miscarriage, you'll be surprised by the enormity of your grief.

Like millions of women, you may recognize the developing fetus as an integral part of yourself from the earliest stages of pregnancy.[203] Researchers L. G. Peppers and R. J. Knapp found no differences in the intensity or patterns of grief among women who miscarried versus those experienced stillbirth or neonatal death.

Your loss may feel so painful because there's an immediate psychological bonding between a mother and her fetus. "The major changes in a woman's hormonal makeup take place early in pregnancy, almost just after conception," writes Jonathan Scher, M.D., author of *Preventing Miscarriage: The Good News*. "Mothers undergo huge hormonal fluctuations and we tend to think this grows along with her swelling belly. But in fact the greatest impact occurs early in pregnancy. So when you lose a pregnancy, there is scientific (hormonal) proof that these feelings occur."

In an attempt to avoid the pain, many women struggle not to grieve over a miscarriage, but as we stressed earlier, it's vital for emotional recovery and growth to fully mourn such a profound loss. Only when we allow ourselves to feel pain and share our grief with those we trust are we able to begin the healing process.

If you've miscarried, especially if it was early on, it can be tempting to rush ahead with the next treatment cycle. However, losing a baby is a big deal, and you need to treat it with the respect you and your unborn child deserve. It's crucial that you're kind and nurturing toward yourself at this time and avoid any situations that are going to cause pain (such as baby showers). Give yourself the time and space to grieve and to accept and experience all your feelings.

Grief isn't something you can run away from—in fact, it's been observed in women 20 years after their miscarriage.[204] Don't be surprised if you feel a huge sense of guilt and self-blame and worry that you miscarried because of something you did, such as riding a bike. It can't be stressed enough that miscarriage isn't your fault, but when you're in pain and desperate to find answers, you may blame yourself or even your doctor or fertility clinic.

Visualization for Healing Self-Blame

Sit comfortably and close your eyes. Breathe deeply and release all the stress you can. Imagine that you're sitting near the ocean as a bright light shines on you and sucks out any tension that's left. The only weight you still have is a bag on your back that the light cannot penetrate. This bag is filled with self-blame and anger. Feel its weight as you walk toward the ocean. Take the bag off your back, open it, and pull out the blaming words and phrases. Repeat them out loud as you throw them one by one into the ocean— hurl them like heavy stones into the sea. Watch the tide carry away your self-blame, and then imagine walking back, feeling stronger and lighter with every step.

Freeing yourself from such negative feelings can add to your sense of closure and may also contribute to the success of future treatments, if you decide that's what you want to do. In a study of 195 couples with a history of recurring miscarriage, researchers found that among women who were involved in emotional recovery programs, 85 percent conceived again, while of those in the control group, only 35 percent had successful pregnancies.[205]

What's more, if you have unresolved grief, this may stop you from fully experiencing the joy of any future pregnancy. "If you feel that you haven't fully grieved over a miscarriage," says Niravi Payne, founder of the Whole Person Fertility Program in New York, "I recommend that you express what you're feeling—verbally or nonverbally—by engaging in some form of grief ceremony." This can be a funeral, a letter you write to your unborn child, saying a prayer, or recording your experiences in a diary. The important thing is to acknowledge your grief.

Secondary Infertility

> *"Every time a treatment failed, people kept telling me, 'Never mind, you already have a child,' and I'd say to them, 'Look, I don't want to be reassured—I just want to tell you that I know I have a lovely daughter already, but I want another child so badly.'"* — Sylvia, 38 years old

Just because you've been pregnant once doesn't always a guarantee that you will be again, especially if PCOS is involved, since it decreases your chances of conceiving. Secondary infertility—the inability to conceive by women who already have one biological child—isn't as rare as it sounds, and the condition is even more common statistically than primary infertility (those who've never been able to have a child).

According to the National Center for Health Statistics, more than half of American women who couldn't conceive or carry a baby to term already had at least one child; other estimates are as high as 70 percent.

Couples with this problem are often assumed to be fertile because they've succeeded in the past, and as a result, they're only half as likely to seek medical treatment. But if you want another child and have PCOS, don't assume that the second time around won't be a problem. It isn't a good idea to delay treatment since we've seen how PCOS can negatively impact your chances.

The Links with PCOS

Why is PCOS linked to secondary infertility? If you've gained weight from your first baby, rather than lost it, can this make your symptoms worse? Or is it because you're a stressed working mom and it's put you under a lot of pressure? The feelings of couples unable to have more than one child are often slighted, and if this is your situation, you may find that your position creates jealousy rather than solidarity with those who are child free and infertile. Since you succeeded once before, people tend to feel that your disappointment isn't as great, but this simply isn't the case.

"Secondary infertility hurts—you may be surprised how much. You probably never anticipated that the inability to complete your desired family could cause such pain," says Massachusetts infertility therapist and support-group leader for RESOLVE, Harriet Fishman Simons. "The sense of failure and anguish is just as deep as for the woman who never gives birth, because they feel the loss of their dream of a larger family."

"I've always dreamed of having four children, a couple dogs, and a house with a large yard for the kids to play in. That dream might never come true now . . . and my throat hurts and my eyes well up with tears whenever I think of it." — Marina, 39 years old

Treatment in these cases would be no different than for primary infertility, and therapy should also be along the same lines. It involves acknowledging grief, managing stress productively, learning new coping skills, and gathering support.

A Different Life

You may not be able to see it at the moment, but there are compensations for being child free. When you feel ready, you can begin to concentrate on these advantages, the most significant being your freedom—the ability to pursue your interests, career or vocation, and to live your life the way you choose. Perhaps you'll travel, work with children in another capacity, or find other ways to mother. You can nurture siblings, friends, parents, other people, ideas, communities, projects, jobs, plants, animals, and so on. Whatever you decide, nothing will be as tough as the endless cliff-hanger of infertility treatment.

"There are infinitely more ways to lead a meaningful, successful life than by becoming a parent," says family therapist Beverly Engel, who practices in Cambria, California. "Child-free living need not be merely tolerated, but can be a positive, fulfilling, and joyous experience."

Your situation doesn't mean that you aren't able to include other children in your life. You can make an incredible impact on their lives by teaching, mentoring, and being a role model. There are opportunities to befriend and tutor children, sponsor a child in another country, work with young people in a professional and volunteer capacity, act as a godparent or caretaker for your friends and family, and so on.

There are so many contributions necessary for a child's development that you don't have to look far to find someone who can benefit from your time and attention, and you should never underestimate the impact you can have. It's high time that we begin to value these contributions as highly as the birthing experience.

"I look back now at the anguish of every month that periods arrived without any respect for my feelings, and I remember my overwhelming desire to be a mom—and I can't believe we got through it and came out the other side. After a lot of talking with each other and with my PCOS sisters online, we finally made the decision not to put ourselves through this anymore.

"It still hurts to think that we can't have kids who will share our genetic heritage—but then, maybe it's a blessing that I won't be passing on PCOS to a biological daughter. Instead, I can bring all my mothering skills, and my husband can bring all of his fathering skills, into the lives of our nieces and nephews and the kids at the playgroup where I finally got the courage to work. It's a different way to be a mom, but I'm getting so much out of it."
— Dionne, 42 years old

Shaping a successful social life can be hard if you're surrounded by people with children, and many friends drift apart when one has kids and the other doesn't. If this is the case, and you can't find common ground, then you need to seek out friends who are also child free. Look for those who are living happy and positive lives and get to know them. In order to do that, you need to get involved in activities that aren't child centered, such as discussion groups, travel clubs, and so on.

Let people know that you want to meet other child-free people, and you'll find lots of them, so there's no need to feel alone. The number of women in this situation is increasing every year, and the U.S. now has a child-free network with more than 50 places to meet. (See the Resource Guide for details.)

Bringing Children into Your Life

If you feel that you want to experience mothering even though you can't carry a child yourself, and you and your partner agree that this is something you both want to explore, then adoption and foster parenting can offer you the chance to do so.

Adoption

"I don't think I could have gotten through this whole PCOS-infertility nightmare without the knowledge that adoption was a possibility. We just felt that we had so much love to give, and after six years of infertility treatment, we began to accept that maybe our role was to do that in another way. I had to work hard and fight every inch of the way, but eventually we became the proud parents of our—and I mean 'our' in every sense of the word—adopted sons. From the moment I saw them at five months old, they were my babies—my long-awaited children."
— Anna, 34 years old

If you consider adoption, you'll find that you need to go through a barrage of assessments that can be daunting, stressful, and frustrating. Most adoption agencies will only consider your application when you've completely given up on fertility treatments, primarily to ensure that you've come to terms with your infertility.

Agencies expect both partners to be in reasonably good health, and your social background will be taken into account. Most will look at your income, so you'll need to demonstrate that you can materially care for a child. Adoption demands a lot from you and your partner, and you both need to appear committed and positive in front of everyone involved. It can be tough and time consuming—but then, so can fertility treatment, and if you really want to give a child a warm, loving home, it's worth looking into this option.

Research has shown that contrary to some people's fears, adopted children turn out to be well adjusted and stable, and the process has no negative effects at all on intelligence. "Obviously all parents—both fertile and infertile—worry about how their children will develop," says fertility expert Robert Winston. "There is not the slightest evidence that adopted children are worse off."

Adopted children have the right and the need to know that they're adopted, and you must be ready to deal with their desire to discover their past at some point. This shouldn't create long-term difficulties since the nurturing aspect of parenthood has a far greater impact than the biological. If they do want to make contact with their birth family, know that the curiosity is natural and doesn't reflect on you as adoptive parents or your relationship with the children.

If you think that you'd like to adopt, the first thing to do is contact your nearest adoption agency (see the Resource Guide for details). You have the best chance if you're in a relationship and are 21–35 years old (21–40 for the man), but because of the surplus of children with special needs, the rules will become far more flexible for those children, allowing single women and older couples better opportunities.

There are no guarantees that you'll be matched with a child, and even if it does fall into place, it's still hard work that's never going to go away. Adoption isn't for everyone: It has its challenges as well as joys, and not every couple will feel emotionally equipped to deal with it, but if you decide that it's right for you, it could turn out to be one of the best decisions you ever made.

Foster Parenting

In many ways, fostering is no different than adoption. You take care of a child's emotional, physical, social, and educational needs on a daily basis. The only difference is that in this case, you don't become legal parents and may also share responsibility with the birth parents.

Children who need foster care are those who, for whatever reason, are vulnerable in their home environment. The family unit may have broken down, or there may be learning difficulties or a disability. Whatever the reason, the birth parents are in crisis and can't cope alone, so the local authorities step in and help the family sort out its problems and develop strategies for the child's future.

Applying to become a foster parent involves a lot of paperwork and assessment by social workers. You may also need to undergo a short period of training, since it's likely that many of the children will be troubled or confused.

Foster parents can feel powerless since they have few legal rights over the child, and they may also be vulnerable to allegations of abuse because many of the children will be emotionally damaged. You may long to bond with foster children, but at the end of the day, you know that they can be returned to their birth parents at any minute, which can stop you from becoming too attached. Fostering requires great strength of mind, stamina, and compassion. (For more information see the Resource Guide.)

Mentoring

In the U.S., there are lots of opportunities to get involved in the lives of children if adoption doesn't work out. You could offer support and inspiration to a disadvantaged child by becoming a mentor or joining the Big Brothers Big Sisters of America (see the Resource Guide), or get involved in a program through your local school district, house of worship, or community center.

Final Reminders for Infertile Couples

Every couple must find their own way to cope with being child free, but here are some general points that may help if you have PCOS and have been told no further treatment is possible:

1. **Allow yourself to mourn.** Being told you're infertile is a bitter blow. You may feel that the pain is something you'll never get over, but the healing process can only begin when you grieve and really cry. Give yourself the time, the space, and the right to mourn. Only when you do so can you begin to deal with the situation and live again.

2. **Stop worrying about the past.** It doesn't help to think about how you postponed the baby decision too long, to dwell on an abortion you had that was necessary in a different situation, or to be upset that you didn't seek help for PCOS earlier. You had your reasons, and there's no point in dwelling on "what if" scenarios.

3. If PCOS contributed to your infertility, **don't blame yourself** and stop feeling guilty. PCOS isn't your fault, and neither is the fact that you can't get pregnant. "In my experience," says Robert Winston, "infertility is never anyone's fault—just as catching influenza or developing cancer is no one's fault."

4. **Accept that you've tried your best.** If you don't think you did all that you could, have the courage to face that fact and acknowledge the reasons why.

5. **Don't let your feelings take over your life** or dominate your relationships with friends and family. While it's good to be open with those who care about you, continually referring to the situation may be difficult for some of your friends to cope with.

6. **Don't be seduced by "wonder cures."** Infertility treatment sells newspapers, so ignore all those sensational headlines about new therapies or women who give birth in their 60s. Remain healthily skeptical about overoptimistic success rates reported in the press.

7. **Communicate with your partner**—he's likely to be your biggest supporter. Figure out how you can spend more times doing things together, and discuss how you can make sex a pleasure again, rather than a baby-making process. Infertility has many destructive effects on couples, but it can also strengthen and improve them. Do your best to enhance the positive aspects of your relationship and your life.

8. **Join a support group** for people who are child free (see the Resource Guide).

9. **Choose your language carefully**—it can be powerful. Therefore, it's important to decide on the term you wish to use for your status regarding infertility. Some people prefer the term *child free* to *childless* because the latter connotes incompleteness, a loss of some sort, or deficiency. If you've been trying to have a baby for some time, you may not feel free at all, but you do at least have the option to live child free instead of continuing to fight a losing battle—you have the choice to stop your treatments and experience a different way of life.

10. Ask yourself whether or not you have the chance to **develop other aspects of your life.** If you aren't bringing up children, you'll probably have more time and freedom than parents do. Perhaps you could put more into your job. Hobbies, home decorating,

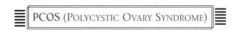

friendships, family, travel, and volunteer work are other areas where many child-free women find ways to make radical changes in their lives and impart great benefits to the lives of others.

   11. **Remember that *all* life choices bring compromise.** Try to keep in mind that motherhood, as rewarding and as absorbing as it is, is a phase—like studying for an exam or doing a big research project. It does, of course, start a lifelong relationship, but so does having a best friend, lover, or sibling.

   Life is about more than just raising children, and everyone discovers this—even mothers, when their children finally leave home. It's just something that those without kids learn earlier. Sure, child-free women miss out on some things, but nobody can have everything, including parents. After all, they spend a lot of their lives tired, anxious, or preoccupied. When one door is closed, no amount of anger or tears will change that, but other doors will open. Why not see what options and possibilities lie ahead?

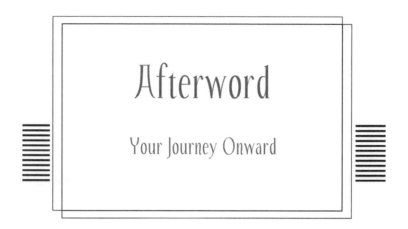

Afterword

Your Journey Onward

You may decide that you want to try to have a baby now or sometime in the future or that children aren't for you. You may get pregnant easily, have to enlist the support of medical technology, or decide that adoption or fostering are good choices in your situation. You may have to struggle to get the treatment you want and need.

Whatever path lies ahead, reading about the options and possibilities available will reduce your feelings of vulnerability so that you feel more in charge, informed, and able make decisions that work for you.

There are three things that we hope you'll take away with you after reading this book:

1. **Getting informed is the best way to feel more in control,** and in addition to reading this book, you can do so by talking to your doctor and other women with PCOS.

"Trying to get my doctor to give me information was like banging my head against a brick wall, but when I found other women over the Internet who were sharing lots of tips and advice they'd gotten from their doctors or specialists, it made me feel much better and more in control. I realized that I wasn't 'infertile—end of discussion,' and that there were options like Clomid

and metformin to help me out. That gave me the boost I needed to decide I'd try to get pregnant because it took away my sense of loneliness and fear of the unknown. And after nearly two years of trying on our own and then deciding to get help, the Clomid worked, and I'm expecting a baby." — Patricia, 34 years old

"Just finding out from my specialist that many women with PCOS become moms took the pressure off me. When I first got diagnosed at the age of 26, I was told that I should really be think-ing about kids, given my condition . . . and I'm sure my desper-ation showed through and put off all the guys I was dating! When I finally got the information I needed, I felt much more relaxed. Now I have a special person in my life and, well, I'm finally happy to wait and see what happens next!" — Sherie, 28 years old

2. **Taking care of yourself is well worth the effort** because changing you and your partner's diet and lifestyle can make a big difference in your chances of conceiving with PCOS. It might sound really simple, but it's powerful and something that's within your control every day.

"My daughter, Noa, was born in October 2003 after a straighforward pregnancy and natural labor. I followed the <u>PCOS Diet Book</u> guidelines prior to getting pregnant and as much as pos-sible after conceiving, and I'm sure they helped me feel great the entire time. Learning how important diet is when you've got PCOS really focused me on what I could do to help myself. Two of my friends with PCOS have also just had babies after making those diet and lifestyle changes." — Eve

"I couldn't believe that seeing a nutritionist could make such a difference in my life! I felt so stressed out and depressed about not getting pregnant, and a friend of mine recommended this idea since it had cured her PMS. So I went to find out more about getting my health back on track through eating well; I was determined to do something positive for myself after spending so much time putting myself down for 'failing.'

"It sounds silly, but nourishing myself with good food and taking the time to see my body as my friend, not my enemy, gave me a whole new supply of energy to try for a baby again. And it gave our relationship a new zing because my bad moods had ended, and I remembered that being in love with this wonderful man was the reason I wanted to have a baby in the first place. We're trying for our second child now, and I'd recommend a self-care program to anyone." — Heather, 37 years old

3. Finally, **ask for support** from other women and their partners who are dealing with PCOS. It can be a really fantastic experience—there's nothing quite like being able to talk or e-mail with someone who knows what you're going through, and who might even have a few new ideas to help you on your PCOS fertility journey.

"The hardest thing for me about having PCOS is thinking about whether I want to have kids or not. At the moment, I just don't know, and I really don't want PCOS to make me panic. I'd say this to every woman out there in the same situation that I am: Talk to each other through support groups, and talk to your husbands and families—the more talking you do, the clearer it gets." — Gaby, 31 years old

And knowing how much help it can be to get that support, we'd love to ask you to offer it, too, if you're ever in a position to do so. After all, the more women with PCOS who ask questions, share stories, and talk about what has worked for them to boost fertility, the more we'll be able to contribute when we see our doctors and specialists, and the better treatment we—and the women who come after us—will get. Every little bit helps—just anonymously posting your story on a support-group Website will hit home for someone out there who's been feeling the same way and wishing someone else knew what it was like. You really can touch the lives of other women going through their PCOS fertility journeys, as well as taking charge of your own.

We hope this book has helped you on your way.

APPENDIX

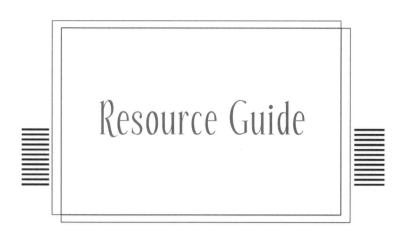

Resource Guide

If you want to find out more about PCOS in general, meet other women dealing with fertility issues, or find out more about women's fertility, following are some of the best and most relevant contacts, books, and Websites. Remember, the beauty of the Internet is that it's international, so you can get some great help and information from any of the Websites listed here, not just from groups based in your country. If you do write to an organization, always send a self-addressed, stamped envelope (SASE), since many of these places are charities and run by volunteers.

In addition to your doctor's advice, a PCOS support group should be your first port of call. Groups such as PCOS Support in the U.S. can help put you in touch with a local organization and also give you the advice, help, and information you need to make informed choices about PCOS and your fertility.

United States

PCOS

Polycystic Ovarian Syndrome
Association Inc. (PCOSA)
P.O. Box 80517
Portland, OR 97280
(877) 775-PCOS
www.pcosupport.org

PCOTeen (A division of PCOSA)
**www.pcosupport.org/pcoteen/
about.html**

Soul Cysters (PCOS-support Website)
www.soulcysters.com
Online support and a place
to share PCOS histories

Adoption, Fostering, and Mentoring

National Council for Adoption
1930 17th Street, NW
Washington, D.C. 20009
(202) 328-1200
www.ncfa-usa.org
National Foster Care Association
www.nfpainc.org

National Council for
Single Adoptive Parents
P.O. Box 15084
Chevy Chase, MD 20815
(202) 966-6367
www.adopting.org

Adoptive Families of America, Inc.
2309 Como Avenue
St. Paul, MN 55108
(800) 372-3300
www.adoptivefam.org

National American Council
on Adoptable Children
970 Raymond Avenue, Suite 106
St. Paul, MN 55114-1149
(651) 644-3036
www.nacac.org

One to One
(Information for adults interested
in being mentors.)
2801 M Street NW
Washington, D.C. 20007
(202) 338-3844
www.mentoring.org

Big Brothers Big Sisters of America
(Information for adults interested
in being mentors.)
230 North 13th Street
Philadelphia, PA 19107
(215) 567-7000
www.bbbsa.org

Biological-Clock Anxiety

Single Mothers by Choice
or Chance
P.O. Box 1642
Gracie Square Station
New York, NY 10028
(212) 988-0993
www.singlemothers.org

RESOLVE
1310 Broadway
Somerville, MA 02144-1731
(617) 623-0744
www.resolve.org

American Association
of Marriage and Family Therapists
1133 15th Street NW, Suite 300
Washington, D.C. 20005
(800) 374-2638
www.aamft.org

Concerned Counseling
(888) 415-8255
http://concernedcounselling.com

Complementary Therapies

National Clearing House for Complementary and Alternative Medicine
P.O. Box 8218
Silver Spring, MD 20907-8218
(888) 664-6226
www.nccam.nih.gov

Harvard University's Mind/Body
Center for Women's Health
The Mind/Body Program for Infertility
(617) 632-9530 or (617) 632-9543
www.mindbody.harvard.edu

Niravi Payne
Whole Person Fertility Program
100 Remson Street
Brooklyn, NY 11201
(800) 666-HEALTH
Phone consultations: (941) 472-7792
www.niravi.com

Joan Z. Borysenko, Ph.D.
Mind-Body Health Sciences, Inc.
393 Dixon Road
Boulder, CO 80302
(303) 440-8460
www.joanborysenko.com

Diabetes

National Diabetes Information
Clearing House (NDIC)
1 Information Way
Bethesada, MD 20892-3560
(301) 654-3810
www.diabetes.org

Diabetes links
www.mendosa.com/org.htm

Eating Disorders

National Eating Disorders Association
603 Stewart St., Suite 803
Seattle, WA 98101
(206) 382-3587
www.nationaleatingdisorders.org

Eating Disorder Recovery
(888) 520-1700
www.edrecovery.com

Fertility and Preconceptual Care

The Fertility Institute
6020 Bullard Avenue
New Orleans, LA 70128
(800) 375-0048
www.fertilityinstitute.com

American Fertility Society (AFS)
2140 11th Avenue South, Suite 200
Birmingham, AL 53205-2800
(205) 933-8484
*Other fertility information
and support Websites:*
www.preconception.com
www.obgyn.net

Infertility

American Infertility Association
666 Fifth Avenue, Suite 278
New York, NY 10103
(718) 621-5083
www.americaninfertility.org

American Society
for Reproductive Medicine
409 12th Street S.W., Suite 203
Washington, D.C. 20024-2125
(202) 863-2439
www.asrm.org
(Offers listings of infertility support
groups, surrogacy and egg donor
programs, and reproductive specialists
by state, plus other information.)

National Infertility
Network Exchange
P.O. Box 204
East Meadow, NY 11554
(516) 794-9772
www.nine-infertility.org

International Council of Infertility
Information Dissemination
P.O. Box 91363
Tuscon, AZ 91363
(520) 544-9548
www.inciid.org

RESOLVE
The National Infertility Association
1310 Broadway Avenue
Somerville, MA 02144
(617) 623-0744
www.resolve.org

The Child-Free Network
6966 Sunrise Blvd, Suite 111
Citrus Heights, CA 95610

Miscarriage

A.M.E.N.D.
4324 Berrywick Terrace
St. Louis, MO 63128
(314) 487-7528

SHARE (Pregnancy and infant-loss
support group)
St. Joseph's Health Center
300 First Capital Drive
St. Charles, MO 63301
(314) 947-6164
www.nationalshareoffice.com

Support group listings:
**www.kumc.edu/gec/
support/miscarri.htmi**

Nutrition

American Academy of Nutrition
College of Nutrition
3408 Sausalito
Corona del Mar, CA 92625-1638
(949) 760-6788
www.nutritioneducation.com

Food and Nutrition
Information Center
National Agriculture Library
10301 Baltimore Avenue, Room 30
Beltsvile, MD 20705-2351
(301) 504-5719
www.nal.usda.gov

Women's Health

National Women's
Health Resource Center
120 Albany Street, Suite 820
New Brunswick, NJ 08901

(877) 986-9742
www.healthywoman.org

Christiane Northrup, M.D.
Health Wisdom for Women
Philips Publishing, Inc.
P.O. Box 60042
7811 Montrose Road
Potomac, MD 20859-0042
(800) 221-8561

United Kingdom

PCOS

Verity
The Graystone Center
28 Charles Square
London NI 6HT
www.verity-pcos.org.uk

Adoption and Fostering

Adoption Information Line
193 Market Street
Hyde
Cheshire SK14 1HF
0800 793 4086
www.adoption.org.uk

British Agencies for Adoption
and Fostering (BAAF)
Skyline House
200 Union Street
London SE1 OLX
020 7593 2000
www.baaf.org.uk

Adoption U.K.—Advice and support
Manor Farm
Appletree Road
Chipping Warden, Banbury
Oxfordshire
OX17 1LH
0870 7700 450
www.adoptionuk.org

National Foster Care Association
(NFCA)
Leonard House
517 Marshalsea Road
London SE1 1EP

020 7357 8015
www.epolitix.com

Overseas Adoption Helpline
First Floor, 34 Upper Street
London N1 OPN
020 7226 7666

Gay and Lesbian Foster
Carers Association
c/o London Friend
86 Caledonian Road
London N1 9DN
020 8854 8888 x2088

Biological-Clock Anxiety

British Association for Counselling
1 Regent Place
Rugby
Warwickshire CV 21 2PJ
01788 550899/578328
www.bac.co.uk

Exploring Parenthood
4 Ivory Place
Treadgold Street
London W11 4BP
020 7221 6681

Family Planning Association
2-12 Pentonville Road
London N1 9FP
020 7837 5432
www.fpa.org.uk

Relationship Guidance

Relate
Herbert Gray College
Little Church Street
Rugby CV21 3AP
01788 573241
www.relate.org.uk

Complementary Therapies

Alternative Health Information Bureau
01923 469 495

Center for the Study of
Complementary Medicine
01703 334752

British Holistic Medical Association
59 Lansdown Place
Hove, East Sussex BN3 1FL
01273 725951
www.bhma.org.uk

British Complementary Medicine
Association
249 Fosse Road
Leicester LE3 1AE
0116 282 5511
www.bcma.uk

National Institute
of Medical Herbalists
56 Longbrook Street
Exeter
Devon EX4 6AH
01392 426022
www.nimh.org.uk

Register of Chinese Herbal Medicine
020 8904 1357
www.rchm.co.uk

British Homeopathic Association
27a Devonshire Street
London W1N 1RJ
020 7935 2163
www.trusthomeopathy.org

Society of Homeopaths
01604 621400
www.homeopathy-soh.org

British Acupuncture Council
Park House
206-8 Latimer Road
London W10 6RE
020 8735 0400
www.acupuncture.org

British Hypnotherapy Association
020 7723 4443
www.hypnotherapy-uk.org

Aromatherapy Organizations Council
P.O. Box 355
Croydon CR9 2QP
020 8251 7912
www.aocuk.net

International Federation
of Aromatherapists
020 8742 2605
www.int-fed-aromatherapy.co.uk

International Federation
of Reflexologists
020 8667 9458
www.reflexology-ifr.com

Association of Reflexologists
27 Old Gloucester Street
London WCIN 3XX
08705 673320
http://www.aor.org.uk
www.aor.org.uk

Transcendental Meditation
Beacon House
Willow Walk, Woodley Park
Skelmersdale
Lancs WN8 6UR
08705 143733

General Council and Register
of Naturopaths
Frazer House
6 Netherhall Gardens
London NW3 5RR
0207 435 6464
www.naturopathy.org.uk

Also:
Michelle Roques-O'Neil at
www.purealchemy.co.uk

Reflexologist Jacqui Garnier
at Garnier70@aol.com

Diabetes

British Diabetic Association
10 Queen Anne Street
London W1M OBD
020 7323 1531
www.diabetes.org.uk

Eating Disorders

Eating Disorders Association
Sackville Place
44 Magdalen Street

Norwich, Norfolk NR3 1JE
0160 362 1414
www.edauk.com

Overeaters Anonymous
01273 624712
Local groups throughout the U.K.
www.oagb.org.uk

Fertility and Pre-conceptual Care

ISSUE: The National Fertility
Association
114 Lichfield Street
Walsall WS1 1SZ
01922 722888
www.issue.co.uk

National Childbirth Trust
Alexander House
Oldham Terrace
Acton, London W3 7NH
www.nct-online.org

Foresight: Association for the
Promotion of Pre-conceptual Care
28 The Paddock
Godalming
Surrey GU7 1XD
01483 427839
www.foresight-preconception.org.uk

Maternity Alliance
Third Floor West
2-6 Northborough Street
London EC1V OAY
0207 490 7638
www.maternityalliance.org.uk

www.fertilityuk.org
A great fertility website that
promotes fertility awareness.

Dr. Sarah Temple at
www.privatefamilydoctor.com.

Infertility Support

Human Fertilization and Embryo
Authority (HFEA)
(Publishes a patient guide to

infertility clinics around the
country, with success rates.)
Paxton House
30 Artillery Lane
London E1 7LS
020 7377 5077
www.hfea.gov.uk

CHILD: National Infertility
Support Network
Charter House
43 St. Leonards Road
Bexhill on Sea
East Sussex TN40 1JA
01424 732361
www.child.org.uk

British Infertility Counselling
Association
69 Division Street
Sheffield S1 4GE
01342 843880
www.bica.net

Infertility Support Group
c/o Women's Health
52 Featherstone Street
London EC1Y 8RT
020 7251 6580
www.womens-health.co.uk

More-to-Life (U.K.-based child-free
network)
114 Lichfield Street
Walsall
WS1 1SZ
070 500 37905
www.moretolife.co.uk

Miscarriage

Miscarriage Association
c/o Clayton Hospital
Northgate
Wakefield
West Yorks WF1 3JS
01924 200 799
www.miscarriageassociation.org.uk

Miscarriage support group listings:
**www.kumc.edu/gec/support/
miscarri.html**

Nutrition

British Association of Nutritional
Therapists
27 Gloucester Street
London WIN 3XX
0870 6061284
www.bant.org.uk

Women's Nutritional Advisory Service
01273 487366
www.wnas.org.uk

Women's Health

Women's Health
52 Featherston Street
London EC1Y 8RT
020 7251 6580
www.womens-health.co.uk

For information about self-insemina-
tion and UK clinics that don't discrimi-
nate against single women or
lesbians, contact Rights of Women
(same address, 020 7251 6577) or
Lesbian Parenting (same address,
020 7251 6576).

Australia

PCOS

POSAA: Polycystic Ovary Syndrome
Association of Australia
P.O. Box E140
Emerton NSW 2770
61 2 4733 4342
www.posaa.asn.au

Adoption

Adoption and Permanent Care Service
Department of Community Services
Level 9, Signature Tower
2-10 Wentworth Street
Parramatta NSW 2150
61 2 8855 4900
**www.community.nsw.gov.au/
adoptions/**

Alternative Therapies

Australasian Integrative Medicine
Association
Locked Bag 29
Clayton VIC 3168
Australia
61 3 9594 7561
www.aima.net.au

Nutrition

Australasian College of Nutritional
and Environmental Medicine
13 Hilton Street
Beaumaris VIC 3193
61 3 9589 6088
www.acnem.org

Fertility

Fertility Society of Australia
Waldron Smith Management
61 Danks Street
Port Melborune VIC 3207
61 3 9645 6359
www.fsa.au.com

Maternity Coalition
P.O. Box 1190
Blackburn North VIC 3130
www.maternitycoalition.org.au

Infertility

ACCESS: Australia's National
Infertility Network
P.O. Box 959
Parramatta NSW 2124
61 2 9670 2380
www.access.org.au

Suggested Reading

Before You Conceive: The Complete Prepregnancy Guide, John R. Sussmann, M.D. (Bantam Books)
An authoritative and comprehensive guide to boosting your fertility and reducing the risks to your baby before you get pregnant.

Bottle-feeding Without Guilt, Peggy Robin (Prima)

Getting Pregnant: What You Need to Know Right Now, Niels Lauerson, M.D., Ph.D. (Fireside)
Not only addresses the needs of those who are having problems conceiving, but also serves as a guide for anyone planning to have a baby now or in the future.

Help Yourself Cope with Your Biological Clock: How to Make the Right Decision about Motherhood, Theresa Cheung (Hodder and Stoughton)
How to cope positively with biological-clock anxiety.

The Infertility Companion: A User's Guide to Tests, Technology and Therapies, Anna Furse (Thorsons)
Excellent resource for women and couples living in the U.K..

Infertility: The Last Secret, Anna McGrail (Bloomsbury)
Coping with the pain and frustration when you want to have a baby and it just doesn't happen.

In Pursuit of Fertility: A Fertility Expert Tells You How to Get Pregnant, Robert Franklin, M.D. and Dorothy Kay Brockman (Henry Holt)
Dr. Franklin, clinical professor of obstetrics and gynecology at Baylor College of Medicine in Houston, Texas, discusses all the latest medical breakthroughs for treating infertility.

Natural Solutions to Infertility: How to Increase Your Chances of Conceiving and Preventing Miscarriage, Marilyn Glenville, Ph.D. (Piatkus)
Boosting your fertility through diet and lifestyle changes.

PCOS: A Woman's Guide to Dealing with Polycystic Ovary Syndrome, Colette Harris and Dr. Adam Carey (Thorsons)
The first book to discuss PCOS and offer an effective four-point plan to relieve symptoms and improve self-esteem.

The PCOS Diet Book: How You Can Use the Nutritional Approach to Deal with Polycystic Ovary Syndrome, Colette Harris and Theresa Cheung (Thorsons)

Written *by* women with PCOS *for* women with PCOS, this book shows you how to beat the symptoms through diet and lifestyle changes.

PCOS: The Hidden Epidemic, Samuel S. Thatcher, M.D. (Perspective Press)
Dr. Thatcher is a renowned expert in reproductive endocrinology, and this lengthy book, published in 2000, provides a comprehensive overview of PCOS research.

Planning for a Healthy Baby, Belinda Barnes and Suzanne Gail Bradley (Vermillion, in association with Foresight promotion of preconceptual care)
Essential preparation for pregnancy.

The Pregnant Woman's Comfort Book, Jennifer Louden (HarperSanFrancisco)
A self-nurturing guide to your emotional well-being during pregnancy.

Single Mothers by Choice, Jane Mattes (Times Books)
A guide book for single women who are considering, or who have chosen, motherhood.

6 Steps to Increased Fertility, Robert L. Barbieri, M.D.; Alice D. Domar, Ph.D.; and Kevin R. Loughlin, M.D. (Simon and Schuster)
An especially useful book from Harvard Medical School. The step-by-step program uses the best in mind/body medicine to maximize your fertility.

Stay Fertile Longer, Mary Kittel (Pan Macmillan)
Planning for your pregnancy when you're ready—in your 20s, 30s, 40s, or today.

Taking Charge of Your Fertility: The Definitive Guide to Natural Birth Control and Pregnancy Achievement, Toni Weschler (Harper Perennial)
All the information you need to monitor your menstrual cycle—whether to achieve or avoid pregnancy or to just get better control of your moods, your health, and your life.

Wanting Another Child: Coping with Secondary Infertility, Harriet Fishman Simons (Jossey-Blass)
A compassionate resource for couples struggling with secondary infertility.

Weight Management and Fitness Through Childbirth, Theresa Cheung (Hodder and Stoughton)
Everything you need to know about weight management and fitness before, during, and after pregnancy.

What to Expect When You're Expecting, Eilen Eisenberg, Heidi Murkoff (Workman)
The pregnant woman's bible.

The Whole Person Fertility Program: A Revolutionary Mind-Body Process to Help You Conceive, Niravi B. Payne, M.S. and Brenda Lane Richardson (Three Rivers Press)
A mind/body program based on the latest scientific research that helps women and couples discover and work through the emotional barriers to conception.

Women and Self-Esteem: Understanding and Improving the Way We Think and Feel about Ourselves, Linda Sanford (Viking Press, 1985)

Women's Bodies, Women's Wisdom, Christiane Northrup, M.D. (Bantam)
A popular holistic-health guide for women that empowers women to take control of their physical and emotional health.

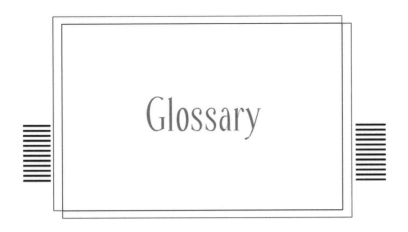

Glossary

Abortion: Pregnancy loss. *Spontaneous abortion* is another name for miscarriage, when the loss has occurred naturally. *Selective abortion* is when the pregnancy, or one or more babies in a multiple pregnancy, is terminated medically.

Acne: Inflammatory condition that affects the sebaceous glands of the skin.

Adrenal gland: Gland that releases DHEA (dehydroepiandrosterone) hormone and other androgens, as well as the stress hormones cortisol and adrenaline.

Alopecia: Hair loss.

Amenorrhea: Absence of menstrual periods.

Amino acids: Building blocks found in proteins that help build, repair, and maintain tissue.

Androgens: Male hormones (such as testosterone, DHEA, and androstendione) responsible for male characteristics, including hair growth, voice change, and muscle development. They're found in both men and women.

Anorexia nervosa: A serious eating dysfunction whereby a person starves him- or herself.

Anovulation: Lack of ovulation or monthly release of an egg from the ovary.

Antiandrogen: Blocks the effects of androgens by blocking the receptor sites or by inhibiting the production of androgens.

Artificial Insemination (AIH): Artificial insemination using the husband or partner's sperm (the "H" in the abbreviation stands for "husband"), introducing it to the cervix by means of a syringe.

Assisted Reproduction (or Assisted Conception): Collective term for infertility treatments.

Assisted Reproduction Technology (ART): Term referring to new medical technologies (including drugs, surgery, micromanipulation, etc.) that aid fertility.

Basal-body temperature (BBT): Temperature of the body at rest.

Blood sugar: Level of glucose present in the bloodstream, used by brain and muscles as energy.

Bulimia: A serious eating dysfunction characterized by bingeing, then purging, often by vomiting or using laxatives.

Cancer: Malignant growth of cells.

Candida albicans: A yeastlike fungus that can be found in the vagina, causing itching, dryness, and discharge; or dryness in the penis. It can also be found in the mouth and the gut.

Carbohydrates: Basic component in food, composed of chains of sugar. Short chains are referred to as *simple carbohydrates* and include table sugar, honey, and fruit sugars. These are converted by the body into glucose, which affects insulin levels. Long chains are called *complex carbohydrates* and include those found in starchy foods such as breads, cereals, potatoes, and vegetables. They are broken down by the body into glucose more slowly than simple sugars, and are either used as immediate energy or are stored by the body for later use.

Cervical mucus: Lubricant secreted by the cervix and vaginal walls that usually changes consistency around ovulation to encourage fertilization.

Cervix: Lowermost part of uterus.

Cesarean section (C-section): Named after Julius Caesar who, according to legend, was born this way, the term refers to surgical delivery of a baby via an incision in the lower abdominal wall, with the mother under local or general anesthetic.

Cholesterol: Waxy substance found in animal fat. In excess, it can contribute to the narrowing of the artery walls, reducing blood flow.

Clomiphene citrate: An ovulation-inducing drug. A popular brand name is *Clomid.*

Conception: The fertilization of an egg by a single sperm.

Congenital: A condition that's present from birth.

Contraception: The prevention of conception with drugs, barrier methods, intrauterine devices (IUDs), or natural methods (herbs, timed intercourse, and so forth).

Corpus luteum: The empty follicle that once held the egg before ovulation; it's responsible for secreting estrogen and progesterone. If fertilization occurs, the corpus luteum sustains the pregnancy until the placenta is formed and takes over.

Cysts: Masses in ovaries that are often filled with fluid; often benign. Can also be found in breasts and elsewhere.

Diabetes: A condition in which the body either does not use insulin efficiently or does not produce insulin at all, resulting in abnormal blood-sugar levels.

Dilation and curettage (D and C): Dilating the cervix and scraping out the lining of the uterus.

Dysmenorrhea: Painful periods.

Ectopic pregnancy: A pregnancy occurring outside the womb. The fertilized ovum attaches itself most commonly in the fallopian tube, but may sometimes stray into the abdominal cavity.

Egg: Female sex cell, also called *ovum, gamete,* and *oocyte.*

Endocrinologist: A specialist of the endocrine system, the body system that controls all hormonal secretion and function.

Endometrium: The lining of the uterus.

Enzymes: Complex proteins found in the bloodstream and tissue.

Estradiol: A naturally occurring estrogen; female hormone.

Estrogen: Female sex hormone produced by the ovary and adrenal gland that causes the development of female characteristics and also plays a role in menstruation and pregnancy.

Fallopian tubes: The part of the woman's reproductive system through which the egg travels to meet the sperm, be fertilized, and then get to the uterus.

Fertilization: Joining of the sperm and egg; the first step in forming an embryo.

Follicle: The sac in the ovary that contains an egg (there are hundreds).

FSH: Follicle-stimulating hormone, which tells the ovary follicle to release an egg each month. (Also the generic name for an ovulation-inducing drug, *Gonal F.*)

Gamete: A sperm or egg.

Gamete intrafallopian transfer (GIFT): Surgical procedure by which sperm and egg are injected directly into a woman's fallopian tubes.

Glucose: Food is digested and converted to glucose, also called *blood sugar;* a source of energy.

Glycemic index: The measure of how a standard number of calories from a food impacts blood sugar when eaten. The faster a food is digested and the more calories it contains, the more the blood-sugar level will spike.

Gonadotropin: Substance that has a stimulating effect on the ovaries or testes.

Gonadotropin-releasing hormone (GnRH): Substance released from the hypothalamus (the part of the brain that controls reproduction) to stimulate the pituitary to produce gonadrotropins, which in turn stimulate the ovary to produce sex steroids.

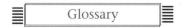

Gonal F: An ovulation-inducing drug; generic name *FSH.*

HCG: Ovulation-inducing drugs pregnyl and profasi; see also *human chorionic gonadotropin.*

High blood pressure: A condition in which the heart pumps blood through the circulatory system at a pressure greater than normal. Normal blood pressure is usually below 140/90mm/Hg. Also called *hypertension.*

Hirsutism: Excess male-type hair growth in women.

Hormone: A chemical substance produced in one organ and carried in the blood to another, where it exerts its effect. An example is FSH, which is produced in the pituitary gland and travels via the blood to the ovaries, where it stimulates the growth and maturation of follicles.

Human chorionic gonadotropin (HCG): Substance derived from the urine of pregnant women. This is what home pregnancy tests detect to confirm pregnancy. Stimulates the corpus luteum of pregnancy to make progesterone.

Human menopausal gonadotropin (HMG): An extract from the urine of menopausal women that contains LH and FSH. Used to stimulate ovulation.

Hyperinsulinism: Elevated insulin levels leading to hypoglycemia.

Hyperthyroidism: Condition characterized by an overactive thyroid gland.

Hypoglycemia: Low levels of blood sugar.

Hypothalamus: A major control center of the brain, which regulates the endocrine and nervous systems. Responsible for maintaining body temperature, sleep, hunger, and reproduction.

Hypothyroidism: Condition characterized by an underactive thyroid gland.

Insulin: A hormone secreted by the pancreas that controls blood-sugar levels. Insulin converts glucose from the bloodstream into glycogen, which is stored in muscle tissue and the liver.

Insulin resistance: Failure of the body to respond properly to the insulin produced by the pancreas. Related to diabetes.

Insulin sensitizers: Group of medications originally used to treat diabetes, but now sometimes used to alleviate many PCOS-related symptoms by helping to correct insulin resistance.

Intrauterine insemination (IUI): Unfrozen, fresh sperm from partner or donor is washed and introduced into the womb via a catheter.

In vitro fertilization (IVF): A process by which an egg is fertilized in the laboratory and then inserted back into the womb.

Laparoscopy: Surgical method involving the use of a tube with a camera on the end, known as a *laparoscope.*

LH: Luteinizing hormone, which is released by the pituitary gland and causes ovulation.

Menopause: When menstruation has stopped for at least one year, usually around age 45–50.

Menses: Monthly discharge of the unfertilized egg and the uterine lining as blood flows through the vagina.

Menstruation: Monthly cycle of hormone production and ovarian activity that prepares the body for pregnancy. If pregnancy doesn't occur, the uterine lining is shed, causing menses.

Metformin: An insulin-sensitizing drug, also known as *glucophage,* which allows the insulin in your body to work more effectively.

Obesity: Abnormal excess of fat, usually defined as more than 20 percent over ideal weight.

Oligomenorrhea: Irregular periods.

Oligozoospermia: Poor sperm count, such as 20 million per ml.

Ovarian hyperstimulation: Rare complication that develops when the ovaries are overstimulated during the use of fertility medications such as Clomid or HMG, then enlarge and produce more follicles. This causes a buildup of fluid in the body, resulting in sudden weight gain, pain in the abdomen, and nausea.

Ovaries: The organs of the female reproductive system that store and release eggs.

Ovulation: The release of an egg from the ovary.

Pancreas: The gland that releases insulin.

Pergonal: An ovulation-inducing drug (generic name is *menotropins*), containing 50 percent FSH and 50 percent LH, to stimulate the ovary to produce eggs. Used in IVF.

Perimenopause: The period of months or years preceding menopause during which time there may be emotional and physical changes, including irregular cycles and fluctuating hormone levels.

Pituitary gland: The gland in the brain that's responsible for regulating hormones associated with milk production and the menstrual cycle.

Placenta: Organ that develops within the uterus during pregnancy. It provides the fetus with nourishment, permits the elimination of waste, and produces hormones needed to sustain the pregnancy.

Postcoital test: A test performed on the sperm and cervical mucus after intercourse to check for mucus hostility and sperm survival.

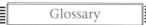

Progesterone: A hormone produced by the corpus luteum in the ovaries, the adrenal gland, and the placenta (in pregnant women). It prepares the uterus for pregnancy and sustains the pregnancy.

Progestin: Name used for certain synthetic or natural progesterone agents. Often contained in birth control pills.

Prolactin: Hormone responsible for milk production.

Prostaglandins: Chemicals that signal the uterine lining to begin shedding.

Proteins: Compounds that contain amino acids. Found in all living matter, proteins are essential for growth and repair of tissue.

Provera: A synthetic progesterone used to treat progesterone deficiency; thickens the lining of the uterus and promote shedding of the endometrium. (Generic name is *metroxyprogesterone.*)

Secondary infertility: Cases of infertility when at least one pregnancy has previously occurred and at least one child has been born.

SHGB: Sex hormone binding globulin.

Sperm count: A measure of a man's fertility that calculates the total number of sperm per ejaculate, as well as that percentage of sperm that are both forward moving (*motility*) and of normal shape and size (*morphology*).

Stein-Leventhal syndrome: The original name for PCOS, named after the two doctors who first diagnosed it.

Subfertility: A state of less than normal fertility.

Testosterone: Male sex hormone responsible for the development of male characteristics.

Test-tube baby: Popular term for a baby fertilized in vitro.

Ultrasound: A diagnostic device that uses sound waves rather than x-rays to visualize the body. Can be done on the abdomen or vaginally.

Unexplained infertility: Cases where no pathology is found in either partner, but pregnancy isn't occurring.

Uterus: The organ of the female reproductive system where the fetus develops.

Zygote: The fertilized ovum; a single fertilized cell resulting from fusion of the sperm and the egg. After further division, the zygote is known as an embryo.

Zygote intrafallopian transfer (ZIFT): A procedure in which a woman's egg is fertilized by her partner's sperm in a petri dish. The resulting zygote is then placed back in her fallopian tube.

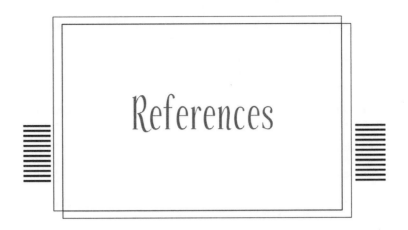

References

1. Trent, M. E., et al. Fertility concerns and sexual behavior in adolescent girls with polycystic ovary syndrome: implications for quality of life. *J Pedatr Adolesc Gynecoll* 2003; 16 (1): 33–7.

2. "Certainly it appears that the risk of miscarriage is increased in mothers with PCOS, as are the risks of gestational diabetes and pregnancy-induced hypertension, unusually small and large babies and C-section rates." From: Thatcher, S. *PCOS: The Hidden Epidemic*. Indianapolis: Perspective Press, 2000 (p. 222).

3. "In conclusion, there are very few women suffering from anovulatory infertility associated with PCOS who cannot be successfully treated today." From: Homburg, R., et al. The management of infertility associated with polycystic ovary syndrome. *Reprod Biol Endocrinol* 2003; 14.

4. Polson, D. W., et al. Polycystic ovaries—a common finding in normal women. *Lancet* 1988; 1: 870–2.

5. Adams, J., et al. Prevalence of polycystic ovaries in women with anovulation and idiopathic hirsuitism. *BMJ* 1986; 293: 355–9.

6. Czeizel, A. E., et al. The effect of preconceptional multivitamin supplementation on fertility. *Int J Vitam Nutr Res* 1996; 66: 55–58.

7. Barnea, E. R., et al. Stress-related reproductive failure. *Journal of In Vitro Fertilization and Embryo Transfer* 1991; 8: 15–23.

8. Swan, S. H., et al. The question of declining sperm density revisited: an analysis of 101 studies published 1934–1996. *Environ Health Perspect* 2000; 108(10): 961–6.

9. Franks, S., et al. The genetic basis of polycystic ovary syndrome. *Hum Reprod* 1997; 12: 2641–8.

10. "Due to the vast array of side effects associated with many pharmaceutical agents typically prescribed to treat PCOS, natural therapies including nutrient supplementation and botanicals may be a less invasive and equally effective approach." From: Marshall, K., et al. Polycystic Ovary Syndrome: clinical considerations. *Alternative Medical Review* 2001; 6(3): 272–92.

11. Richardson, M. R., et al. Current perspectives in polycystic ovary syndrome. *Am Fam Physician* 2003; 68(4): 697–704.

12. Clark, A., et al. Weight loss results in significant improvements in pregnancy and ovulation rates in annovulatory obese women. *Hum Reprod* 1995; 10: 2705–12.

13. Kiddy, D. S., et al. Improvement in endocrine and ovarian function during dietary treatment of obese women with PCOS. *Clin Endocrinol* 1992; 36: 105–11.

14. Cikot, R., et al. Dutch GPs acknowledge the need for preconceptual health care. *Br J Gen Pract* 1999; 49(441): 314.

15. Ontario Early Child Development Research Center. Preconception and Health: Research and strategies: Best start brochure, 2001.

16. Oliva, A., et al. Contribution of environmental factors to the risk of male infertility. *Hum Reprod* 2001; 16(8).

17. Sharpe, R. M., et al. Environment, lifestyle and infertility—an intergenerational issue. *Nat Cell Biol* 2002; 4: s33–40.

18. Bolumar, F., et al. Body mass index and delayed conception: a European Multicenter Study on Infertility and Subfecundity. *Am J Epidemiol* 2000; 151(11): 1072–9.

19. Pasquali, R., et al. Obesity and Reproductive disorders in women. *Hum Reprod Update* 2003; 9(4): 360–70.

20. Hartz, A., et al. The association of obesity with infertility and related menstrual abnormalities in women. *International Journal of Obesity* 1979; 3: 57–73.

21. Alieva, E. A., et al. The effect of a decrease in body weight in patients with the polycystic ovary syndrome. *Akush Ginekol (Mosk)* 1993; 3: 33–6.

22. Foreyt, J. and Poston, W. S. Obesity, a never-ending cycle. *International Journal of Fertility and Women's Medicine* 1998; 48(2).

23. Clark, A. M., et al. Weight loss results in significant improvements in pregnancy and ovulatory rates in annovulatory obese women. *Hum Reprod* 1995; 10.

24. Clark, A. M., et al. Weight loss in obese, infertile women results in improvements in reproductive outcome for all forms of fertility treatment. *Hum Reprod* 1998; 6: 1502–5.

25. Crosignani, P. G., et al. Overweight and obese anovulatory women with polycystic ovaries: parallel improvements and fertility rate induced by diet. *Hum Reprod* 2003; 18(9): 1928–32.

26. Pasquali, R., et al. Obesity and Reproductive Disorders in women. *Hum Reprod Update* 2003; 9 (4): 359–72.

27. Kiddy, D. S., et al. Differences in clinical and endocrine features between obese and non-obese subjects with polycystic ovary syndrome: an anlaysis of 263 cases. *Clin Endocrinol* 1989; 32: 213–20.

28. Robinson, S., et al. Postprandial thermongenesis is reduced in polycystic ovary syndrome and is associated with increased insulin resistance. *Clin Endocrinol* 1992; 36: 537–43.

29. Bray, G., et al. Obesity and Reproduction. *Hum Reprod* 1997; 12(1): 26–32.

30. Moran, L. J., et al. The obese patient with infertility: a practical approach to diagnosis and treatment. *Nutr Clin Care* 2002; 5(6): 290–7.

31. Warren, M. P., et al. The effects of intense exercise on the female reproductive system. *J Endocrinol* 2001; 170(1): 3–11.

32. Holmes, T., et al. Relations of exercise to body image and sexual desirability among a sample of university students. *Psychol Rep* 1994; 74(3 Pt. 1): 920–2.

33. Tyrer, L. B., et al. Nutrition and the Pill. *J Reprod Med* 1984; 547–50.

34. British Medical Association. *Concise Guide to Medicines and Drugs*. London: Dorling Kindersley, 1998; 147.

35. Sozen, I., et al. Hyperinsulinism and its interaction with hyperandrogenism in polycystic ovary syndrome. *Obstet Gynecol Survey* 2000; 55 (5): 321–8.

36. Branigan, E. F., et al. A randomized clinical trial of treatment of clomiphene citrate-resistant anovulation with the use of oral contraceptive pill suppression and repeat clomiphene citrate treatment. *Am J Obstet Gynecol* 2003; 188(6): 1424–8.

37. Spria, N. Fertility of couples following cessation of contraception. *J Biosoc Sci* 1985; 17(3): 281–90.

38. Weisberg, E., et al. Fertility after discontinuation of oral contraceptives. *Clin Reprod Fertil* 1982; 1(4): 261–72.

39. Chasan-Tabar, L., et al. Oral contraceptives and ovulatory causes of delayed fertility. *Am J Epidemiol* 1997; 146(3): 258–65.

40. University of Southern California School of Medicine research study. Mini pill increases risk of diabetes. *J Am Med Assoc*; 1998.

41. Barnea, E. R., et al. Stress-related reproductive failure. *J IVF Embryo Transfer* 1991; 8(1): 15–23.

42. Jakobovits, A. A., et al. Interactions of stress and reproduction. *Zentralbl Gynakol*. 2002; 124(4): 189–93.

43. Lenzi, A., et al. Stress, sexual dysfunctions, and male infertility. *J Endocrinol Invest* 2003; 26(3): 72–6.

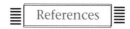

44. Domar, A. D. R., et al. Distress and conception in infertile women: A complementary approach. *J Am Med Wom Assoc* 1999; 45(4).

45. Reiko, K., et al. Work-related reproductive disorders among working women. *Ind Health* 2002; 40: 101–12.

46. Spiegel, K.; Leproult, R.; Van Cauter, E. Impact of sleep on metabolic and endocrine function. *Lancet* 1999; 354: 1435–9.

47. Rice, R., et al. Fish and a healthy pregnancy: more than just a red herring. *Professional Care of Mother and Baby* 1996; 6(6): 171–3.

48. Reece, M. S., et al. Maternal and paternal fatty acids: Possible role in pre-term birth. *Am J Obstet Gynecol* 1997; 176(4): 907.

49. Bayer, R., et al. Treatment of infertility with vitamin E. *Int J Fertil Womens Med* 1960; 5:70–8.

50. Bates, C. J., et al. Plasma carotenoid and vitamin E concentrations in women living in a rural west African (Gambian) community. *Int J of Vitam Nutr Res* 2002; 72(3): 133–41.

51. Rushton, D. H., et al. Ferritin and fertility. *Lancet* 1991; 337: 1554.

52. Rushton, D. H. Ferritin and fertility [letter]. *Lancet* 1991; 337: 1554.

53. Zdziennicki, A., et al. Iron deficiency as a risk factor during the perinatal period. *Ginekol Pol* 1996; 67(6): 301–3.

54. Luck, M. R., et al. Ascorbic acid and fertility. *Biol Reprod* 1995; 52(2): 262–6.

55. Schwabe, J. W. R., et al. Beyond zinc fingers. *Trends in Biochemcial Sciences* 1991; 16: 291–6.

56. Saner, G., et al. Hair manganese concentrations in newborns and their mothers. *Am J Clin Nutr* 1985; 41: 1042–4.

57. Sieve, B. F., et al. The clinical effects of a new B-complex factor, para-aminobenzoic acid, on pigmentation and fertility. *South Med. Surg* 1992; 135–9.

58. Beenet, M., et al. Vitamin B12 deficiency, infertility and recurrent fetal loss. *J Reprod Med* 2001; 46(3): 209–12.

59. Kidd, G. S., et al. The effects of pyridoxine on pituitary hormone secretion in amenorrhea. *J Clin Endocrinol Metab* 1982; 54: 872–5.

60. Crha, I., et al. Ascorbic acid and infertility treatment. *Cent Eur J Public Health* 2003; 11(2): 63–7.

61. Tarin, J., et al. Effects of maternal ageing and dietary antioxidant supplementation on ovulation, fertilisation and embryo development in vitro in the mouse. *Reprod Nutr Dev* 1998; 38(5): 499–508.

62. Battaglia, C., et al. Adjuvant L-arginine treatment for in-vitro fertilization in poor responder patients. *Hum Reprod* 1999; 14: 1690–7.

63. West, K. P., et al. Double-blind cluster randomised trial of low-dose supplementation with vitamin A or beta-carotene on mortality related to pregnancy in Nepal. *BMJ* 1999; 318: 570–5.

64. Rothman, K. J., et al. Teratogenicity of high vitamin A intake. *N Engl J Med* 1995; 333(21): 1369–73.

65. Howard, J. M., et al. Red cell magnesium and glutathione peroxidase in infertile women: Effects of oral supplementation with magnesium and selenium. *Magnes Res* 1994; 7(1): 49–57.

66. Czeizel, A. E., et al. The effect of preconceptional multivitamin supplementation on fertility. *Int J Vitam Nutr Res* 1996; 66: 55–8.

67. Friends of the Earth press briefing for safer chemicals campaign: *Chemicals and Health* **www.foe.co.uk/resource/briefings/chemicals_and_health.pdf**

68. ASH. *Smoking and Reproduction* research studies factsheet, 2000.

69. Baskari, L., et al. Polycyclic aromatic hydrocarbon-DNA adducts in human sperm as a marker of DNA damage and infertility. *Mutat Res* 2003; 535(2): 155–60.

70. Howe, G., et al. Effects of age, cigarette smoking, and other factors on fertility: Findings in a large prospective study. *BMJ* 1985; 290: 1697–9.

71. Weinberg, C. R., et al. Reduced fecundability in women with prenatal exposure to cigarette smoking. *Am J Epidemiol* 1989; 129: 1072–8.

72. Grodstein, F., et al. Infertility in women and moderate alcohol use. *Am J Public Health* 1994; 84: 1429–32.

73. Hatch, E. E. and Bracken, M. B. Association of delayed conception with caffeine consumption. *Am J Epidemiol* 1993; 138: 1082–92.

74. Stanton, C. K. and Gray, R. H. Effects of caffeine consumption on delayed conception. *Am J Epidemiol* 1995; 142: 1322–9.

75. Williams, M. A., et al. Coffee and delayed conception [letter]. *Lancet* 1990; 335: 1603.

76. Wilcox, A., et al. Caffeinated beverages and decreased fertility. *Lancet* 1989; 1(8642): 840.

77. Fenster, L., et al. A prospective study of caffeine consumption and spontaneous abortion. *Am J Epidemiol* 1996; 143(11): 525.

78. Rasch, V., et al. Cigarette, alcohol, and caffeine consumption: risk factors for spontaneous abortion. *Acta Obstet Gynecol Scand* 2003; 82(2): 182–8.

79. Hakim, R. B.; Gray, R. H.; and Zacur, H. Alcohol and caffeine consumption and decreased fertility. *Fertil Steril* 1998; 70 : 632–7.

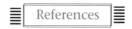

80. Joesoef, M. R., et al. Are caffeinated beverages risk factors for delayed conception? *Lancet* 1990; 335: 136–7.

81. Gerhard, I., et al. Toxic pollutants, solvents and pesticides and fertility disorders. *Geburtshilfe-Frauenheilked* 1993; 53(3): 147–60.

82. Baranski, B. Effects of workplace on fertility and related reproductive outcome. *EnvironHealth Perspect*1993; 101(2): 81–90.

83. Winder, C., et al. Lead, reproduction and development. *Neurotoxicology* 1993; 14: 303.

84. Bogden, J. D., et al. Lead poisoning—One approach to a problem that won't go away. *Environ Health Perspect* 1997; 105(12): 1284–7.

85. Coste, J., et al. Lead-exposed workmen and fertility: A study of 354 subjects. *Eur J Epidemiol* 1991; 7: 154–8.

86. Ward, N., et al. Placental element levels in relation to foetal development of obstetrically normal births: A study of 39 elements. Evidence for effects of cadmium, lead and zinc on foetal growth, smoking as a cause of cadmium. *Int J Biosoc Res* 1987; 9(1): 63081.

87. Gerhard, I., et al. Heavy metals and fertility. *J Toxicol Environ Health* 1998; 54(8): 593–611.

88. Choy, C. M., et al. Infertility, blood mercury concentrations and dietary seafood consumption: a case-control study. *BJOG* 2002 109(10): 1121–5.

89. Rowland, A. S., et al. The effect of occupational exposure to mercury vapor on the fertility of female dentists. *Occup Environ Med* 1994; 51(1): 28–34.

90. Weber, R. F., et al. Male fertility: Possibly affected by occupational exposure to mercury. *Ned Tijdschr Tandheelkd* 2000; 107(12): 495–8.

91. Davies, B. J., et al. Mercury vapor and female reproductive toxicity. *Toxicol Sci* 2001; 59(2): 291–6.

92. Moszczynski, P., et al. Mercury compounds and the immune system: a review. *Int J Occup Med Environ Health* 1997; 10(3): 247–58.

93. Castoldi, A. Neurotoxic and molecular effects of methylmercury in humans. *Rev Environ Health* 2003; 18(1): 19–31.

94. Warfninge, K., et al. The effect of pregnancy outcome and fetal brain development of prenatal exposure to mercury vapor. *Neurotoxicology* 1994; 15(4).

95. Gerhard, I., et al. Heavy metals and fertility. *J Toxicol Environ Health* 1998; 54(8): 593–611.

96. Sharpe, R.M., et al. Environment, lifestyle and infertility—an inter-generational issue. *Nat Cell Biol* 2002; 4: s33–40.

97. Goldhaber, M. K., et al. The risk of miscarriage and birth defects among women who use VDU terminals during pregnancy. *Am J Ind Med* 1988; 13: 695–706.

98. Bramwell, R.S., et al. Visual display units and pregnancy outcome: a prospective study. *J Psychosom Obstet Gynaeco* 1993; 14(3): 197–2.

99. Barnes, J. (In association with FORESIGHT Association for Provision of Pre-conception care) *Planning for a Healthy Baby*. Vermillion Books, 1990: p. 95.

100. Furst, A., et al. Can nutrition affect chemical toxicity? *Int J Toxicol* 2002; 21(5): 419–24.

101. Frisk, P., et al. Selenium protection against mercury-induced apoptosis and growth inhibition in cultured K-562 cells. *Biol Trace Elem Res* 2003; 92(2): 105–14.

102. Patrick, L., et al. Toxic metals and antioxidants: Part II. The role of antioxidants (and zinc) in arsenic and cadmium toxicity. *Altern Med Rev* 2003; 8(2): 106–28.

103. Sanchez-Fructuso, A.L., et al. Lead mobilization during calcium disodium ethylenediaminetetraacetate chelation therapy in treatment of chronic lead poisoning. *Am J Kidney* Dis 2002; 40(1): 51–8.

104. Rabbani, G. H., et al. Antioxidants in detoxification of arsenic-induced oxidative injury in rabbits: preliminary results. *J Environ Sci Health* 2003; 38(1): 273–87.

105. Nazrul Islam, S. K., et al. Serum vitamin E, C and A status of the drug addicts undergoing detoxification: Influence of drug habit, sexual practice and lifestyle factors. *Eur J Clin Nutr* 2001; 55(11): 1022–7.

106. Wang, W., et al. Retinoic acid stimulates annexin-mediated growth plate chondrocyte mineralization. *J Cell Biol* 2002; 10; 157(6): 1061–9. (Epub 2002 Jun 03).

107. Sohlet, A., et al. Blood lead levels in psychiatric outpatients reduced by zinc and vitamin C. *J Orthomolecular Psychiatry* 1977; 6(3): 272–6.

108. Hemingway, R.G. The influences of dietary intakes and supplementation with selenium and vitamin E on reproduction diseases and reproductive efficiency in cattle and sheep. *Vet Res Commun* 2003; 27(2): 159–74.

109. Volesky, B., et al. Bio-sorption of heavy metals. *Biotechnol Prog* 1995; 3(11): 235–50.

110. Quig, D., et al. Cysteine metabolism and metal toxicity. *Altern Med Rev* 1998; 3(4): 262–70.

111. Richmond, V. L. Incorporation of methysulfoneylmethande sulfur into guinea pig serum proteins. *Life Sci* 1986; 39(3): 263–8.

112. Lund, E., et al. Non-nutritive bioactive constituents of plants: dietary sources and health benefits of glucosinolates. *Int J Vitam Nutr Res* 2003; 73(2): 135–43.

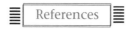

113. Loftus, T., et al. Psychogenic Factors in Anovulatory women: Behavioral and Psychanalytic Aspects of Anovulatory Amenorrhea. *Fertil Steril* 1962; 13: 20.

114. Cutler, W. B., et al. Sexual behavior frequency and biphasic ovulatory type menstrual cycles. *Physiol Behav* 1985; 34(5): 805–10.

115. van Roijen, J. H., et al. Sexual arousal and the quality of semen produced by masturbation. *Hum Reprod* 1996; 11(1): 147–51.

116. Reported in *Psychology Today* (Jan/Feb 1996).

117. Cutler, W. B., et al. Sexual behavior frequency and biphasic ovulatory type menstrual cycles. *Physiol Behav* 1985; 34(5): 805–10.

118. Cossom, J., et al. How spermatozoa come to be confined to surfaces. *Cell Motil Cytoskeleton* 2003; 54(1): 56–63.

119. Richardson, M. R., et al. Current perspectives in polycystic ovary syndrome. *Am Fam Physician* 2003; 15;68(4): 697–704.

120. Shasha, S. M., et al. Morbidity in the ghettos during the Holocaust. *Harefuah* 2002; 141(4): 364–8, 409, 408.

121. Osteria, T. S., et al. Maternal nutrition, infant health, and subsequent fertility. *Philipp J Nutr* 1982; 35(3): 106–11.

122. Milsom, S. R., et al. LH levels in women with polycystic ovarian syndrome: have modern assays made them irrelevant? *BJOG* 2003; 110(8): 760–4.

123. Franks, S. The ubiquituous polycystic ovary. *J Endocrinol* 1991; 129: 317–19.

124. Barbieri, R. L., et al. Hyperinsulinemia and overian hyperandrogenism. *Endocrinol Metab Clin North Am* 1988; 685–703.

125. Richardson, M. R., et al. Current perspectives in PCOS. *Am Fam Physician* 2003; 15 (68): 697–704.

126. Sharpe, R. M., et al. Environment, lifestyle and infertility—an intergenerational issue. *Nat Cell Biol* 2002; 4: s33–40.

127. Moran, L.J., et al. Dietary composition in restoring reproductive and metabolic physiology in overweight women with polycystic ovary syndrome. *J Clin Endocrinol Metab* 2003; 88(2): 812–9.

128. Cassidy, A., et al. Biological effects of a diet of soy protein, rich in isoflavones, on the menstrual cycle of premenstrual women. *Am J Clin Nutr* 1994; 60: 333–40.

129. Aldercreutz, et al. Dietary phytestrogens and cancer. *J Steroid Chem Mol Biol* 1992; 41: 331–7.

130. Auburn, K. J., et al. Indole-3-carbinol is a negative regulator of estrogen. *J Nutr* 2003; 133(7): 2470–7S.

131. Ingram, D. J., et al. *J National Cancer Institute* 1987; 79: 1225.

132. Philips, W. R., et al. Effect of flaxseed ingestion on the menstrual cycle. *J Clin Endocrinol Metabol* 1993; 77(5): 1215–9.

133. Kidd, G. S., et al. The effects of pyridoxine on pituitary hormone secretion in amenorrhea-glactorrhea syndrome. *J Clin Endocrinol Metabol* 1982; 54(4): 872–5.

134. American Diabetics Association. Magnesium supplementation in the treatment of diabetes. *Diabetes Care* 1992; 15: 1065–7.

135. Carranza-Lira, S., et al. The relation of the gonadotrophin response to chlormadinone according to body weight in patients with amenorrhea due to polycystic ovarian syndrome. *Eur J Gynecol Reprod Bio* 1996; 66(2): 161–4.

136. Collins, et al: announced at the 13th International Congress of Dietetics, Edinburgh, Scotland (2000).

137. Hikon, H., et al. Antihepatotoxic actions of flavonolignans from Silybum marianum fruits. *Planta Medica* 1984; 50: 248–50.

138. Clark, A. M., et al. Weight loss results in significant improvements in pregnancy and ovulation rates in annovulatory obese women. *Hum Reprod* 1995; 2705–12.

139. Okajima, T., et al. Hormonal abnormalities were improved by weight loss using very low calorie diet in a patient with polycystic ovary syndrome. *Fukuoka Igaku Zasshi* 1994; 85(9): 263–6.

140. Tolino, A., et al. Obesity and reproduction. *Acta Eur Fertil* 1994; 25(2): 119–21.

141. Barnea, E. R., et al. Stress-related reproductive failure. *J IVF Embryo Transfer* 1991; 8: 15–23.

142. Kaplan, G. Get moving with yoga. *Diabetes Self Management* 2003; 20(4): 28, 31–3.

143. Health benefits of meditation. *Mayo Clin Womens Healthsource* 2003; 7(7): 7.

144. Li, D. J., et al. Summary of National Academic Conference on emmeniopathy and infertility of integrated traditional Chinese and Western medicine. *Zhongguo Zhong Xi Yi Jie He Za Zhi* 2001; 21(3): 238–9.

145. "Due to the vast array of side effects associated with many agents typically used to treat PCOS, natural therapies including supplementation and botanicals may be a less invasive and equally effective approach." From: Marshall, K., et al. PCOS: a clinical consideration. *Altern Med Rev* 2001; 6: 272–92.

146. Czeizel, A. E., et al. The effect of preconceptional multivitamin supplementation on fertility. *Int J Vitam Nutr Res* 1996; 66: 55–8.

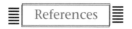

147. Ge, X. L., et al. Treatment of secondary amenorrhea and oligohypomen-orrhea with combined traditional Chinese and Western medicine. *Zhong Xi Yi Jie He Za Zhi* 1991; 11(11): 661–3, 645.

148. Cahill, D. J., et al. Multiple follicular development associated with herbal medicine. *Hum Reprod* 1994; 9(8): 1469–70.

149. Propping, D., et al. Treatment of corpus luteum insufficiency. Zeitschr 1987; 63: 932–3.

150. Sliutz, G., et al. Agnus Castus extract inhibits prolactin secretion of rat pituitary cells. *Horm Metab Res* 1993; 25: 253–5.

151. Jarry, H., et al. In vitro prolactin but not LH and FSH release is inhibited by compounds in extracts of agnus castus: direct evidence for a dopaminergic principle by the dopamine receptor assay. *Exp Clin Endocrinol* 1994; 102(6): 448–54.

152. Gerhard, I., et al. Mastodynon for female infertility: Randomized, placebo-controlled, clinical double-blind study. *Forsch Komplementärmed* 1998; 5: 272–8.

153. Campbell, S. M., et al. Gynecology: select topics. *Prim Care* 2002; 29(2): 297–321.

154. Chaing, H. S., et al. Medicinal plants: Conception/contraception. *Adv Contracept Deliv Syst* 1994; 10(3–4): 355–63.

155. Sakai, A., et al. Induction of ovulation by Sairei-to for PCOS patients. *Endocr J* 1999; 46(1): 217–20.

156. Takahashi, K., et al. Effect of TJ–68 (shakuyaku-kanzo-to) on polycystic ovarian disease. *Int J Fertil Menopausal Stud* 1994; 39(2): 69–76.

157. Pinn, G., et al. Herbal Medicine in Pregnancy Complement. *Ther Nurs Midwifery* 2002; 8(2): 77–80.

158. Ushiroyama, T., et al. Effects of Unikei-to an herbal medicine on endocrine function and ovulation in women with high basal levels of luteinizing hormone secretion. *J Reprod Med* 2001; 46(5): 451–6.

159. Chen, B. Y., et al. Acupuncture normalises dysfunction of hypothalmic-pituitary ovarian axis. *Acupunct Electother Res* 1997; 22 (2): 97–108.

160. Stener-Victorin, E., et al. Effects of electro-acupuncture on anovulation in women with polycystic ovary syndrome. *Acta Obstet Gynecol Scand* 2000; 79 (3): 180–8.

161. Liao, D. L., et al. Influence of artificial cycles induced by traditional Chinese medicine on the releasing and reserving gonadotrophic hormone function of the pituitary gland in the female with secondary amenorrhea. *Zhong Xi Yi Jie He Za Zhi* 1989; 9 (8): 458–61.

162. Gerhard, I., et al. Auricular acupuncture in the treatment of female infertility. *Gynaecol Endocrinol* 1992; 6 (3): 171.

163. Bergman, J., et al. The efficacy of the complex medication Phyto-Hypophyson L in female, hormone-related sterility. A randomized, placebo-controlled clinical double-blind study. *Forsch Komplementarmed Klass Naturheilkd* 2000; 7(4): 190–9.

164. Kaplan, B., et al: Homoeopathy: 2. In pregnancy and for the under-fives. *Prof Care Mother Child* 1994; 4(6): 185–7.

165. Sovino, H., et al. Clomiphene citrate and ovulation induction. *Reprod Biomed Online* 2002; 4(3): 303–10.

166. Sidani, M., et al. Gynecology: select topics. *Prim Care* 2002; 29(2): 297–321.

167. Meirow, D., et al. Ovulation induction in polycystic ovary syndrome: a review of conservative and new treatment modalities. *Eur J Obstet Gynecol Reprod Biol* 1993; 50(2): 123–31.

168. Nasseri, S., et al. Clomiphene citrate in the twenty-first century. *Hum Fertil* 2001; 4(3): 145–51.

169. Haas, D. A., et al. Effects of Metformin on body mass index, menstrual cyclicity, and ovulation induction in women with polycystic ovary syndrome *Fertil Steril* 2003; 79(3): 469–81.

170. Elkind, H., et al. Sequential hormonal supplementation with vaginal estradiol and progesterone gel corrects the effect of clomiphene on the endometrium in oligo-ovulatory women. *Hum Reprod* 2002; 17(2): 295–8.

171. Daimanti-Kandarakis, E., et al. Therapeutic effects of Metformin on insulin resistance and hyperandrogenism in polycystic ovary syndrome 1998; *European J Endocrinol* 1998; 138: 269–74.

172. Morin-Papunen, L. C., et al. Metformin therapy improves the menstrual pattern with minimal endocrine and metabolic effects in women with polycystic ovary syndrome. *Fertil Steril* 69: 691–6.

173. Barbieri, L., et al. Metformin for the treatment of polycystic ovary syndrome. *Obstet Gynecol* 2003; 101(4): 785–93.

174. Stadtmauer, L. A., et al. Should patients with polycystic ovary syndrome be treated with Metformin? Benefits of insulin sensitizing drugs in polycystic ovary syndrome—beyond ovulation induction. *Hum Reprod* 2002; 17(12): 3016–26.

175. Glueck, C. J., et al. Pregnancy outcomes among women with polycystic ovary syndrome treated with Metformin. *Hum Reprod* 2002; 17(11): 2858–64.

176. Tann, S. L., et al. In-vitro maturation of oocytes from unstimulated polycystic ovaries. *Reprod Biomed Online* 2002; 4(1): 18–23.

177. Tiessier, M. P., et al. Comparison of follicle steroidogenesis from normal and polycystic ovaries in women undergoing IVF: relationship between steroid concentrations, follicle size, oocyte quality and fecundability. *Hum Reprod* 2000; 15(12): 2471–7.

178. Diejomaoh, M., et al. The relationship of recurrent spontaneous miscarriage with reproductive failure. *Med Princ Pract* 2003; 12(2): 107–11.

179. Rai, R., et al. Polycystic Ovaries and recurrent miscarriage—a reappraisal. *Hum Reprod* 2000; 15: 612–15.

180. Norman, R. J., et al. Lifestyle factors in the aetiology and management of polycystic ovary syndrome. In: Kovacs, G. (ed.). *Polycysytic Ovary Syndrome* Cambridge: Cambridge University Press, 2000: ch. 9, p. 103.

181. Hamilton, et al. Association of moderate Obesity with a poor pregnancy outcome in women with polycystic ovary syndrome treated with low dose gonadotrophin. *Br J Obstet Gynaecol* 1992; 99: 128–31.

182. Tummers, P., et al. Risk of spontaneous abortion in singleton and twin pregnancies after IVF/ICSI. *Hum Reprod* 2003; 18(8): 1720–3.

183. Ventura, S. J., et al. Highlights of trends in pregnancies and pregnancy rates by outcome: estimates for the United States, 1976–96. *Natl Vital Stat Rep* 1999; 47(29): 1–9.

184. Gupta, S., et al. Polycystic ovarian syndrome: is community care appropriate? *Int J Clin Pract* 1999; 53(5): 359–62.

185. Papp, Z., et al. The evolving role of ultrasound in obstetrics/gynecology practice. *Int J Gynaecol Obstet* 2003; 82(3): 339–46.

186. Turhan, N. O., et al. Assessment of glucose tolerance and pregnancy outcome of polycystic ovary patients. *Int J Gynaecol Obstet* 2003; 81(2): 163–8.

187. Linne, Y., et al. Natural course of gestational diabetes mellitus: long term follow up of women in the SPAWN study. *BJOG* 2002; 109(11): 1227–31.

188. Lepercq, J. The diabetic pregnant woman. *Ann Endocrinol* 2003; 64(3): s7–11.

189. Kasyap, P., et al. Polycystic ovary disease and the risk of pregnancy-induced hypertension. *J Reprod Med* 2000; 45(12): 991–4.

190. Krizanovska, K., et al. Obesity and reproductive disorders. *Sb Lek* 2002; 103(4): 517–26.

191. Wang, J. X., et al. Obesity increases the risk of spontaneous abortion during infertility treatment. *Obes Res* 2002; 10(6): 551–4.

192. Sadrzadeh, S., et al. Birth-weight and age at menarche in patients with polycystic ovary syndrome or diminished ovarian reserve, in a retrospective cohort. *Hum Reprod* 2003; 18(10): 2225–30.

193. Laitinen, J., et al. Body size from birth to adulthood as a predictor of self-reported polycystic ovary syndrome symptoms. *Int J Obes Relat Metab Disord.* 2003; 27(6): 710–5.

194. Jolly, M. C., et al. Risk factors for macrosomia and its clinical consequences: a study of 350,311 pregnancies. *Eur J Obstet Gynecol Reprod Biol* 2003; 111(1): 9–14.

195. Aortsman, J. et al. Gestational diabetes and neonatal macrosomia in the polycystic ovary syndrome. *J Reprod Med* 1991; 36(9): 659–61.

196. Plachot, M., et al. Oocyte and embryo quality in polycystic ovary syndrome. *Gynecol Obstet Fertil* 2003; 31(4): 350–4. Although more oocytes were recovered from PCOS patients, the number of good quality embryos, suitable for transfer or freezing was similar in the two groups as less of the oocytes were mature and the fertilization rate was lower in the PCOS group. IVF or ICSI (according to the indication) are therefore efficient in PCOS patients.

197. Godfrey, K. M., et al. Fetal nutrition and adult disease. *Am J Clin Nutr* 2000; 71(5): 1344–52S.

198. Groenen, P. M., et al. Are myo-inositol, glucose and zinc concentrations in amniotic fluid of fetuses with spina bifida different from controls? *Early Hum Dev* 2003; 71(1): 1–8.

199. Larsen Meyer, D. E., et al. Effect of postpartum exercise on mothers and their offspring: a review of the literature. *Obes Res* 2002; 10(8): 841–53.

200. Connor, C. G., et al. Maternal antenatal anxiety and behavioural/emotional problems in children: a test of a programming hypothesis. *J Child Psychol Psychiatry* 2003; 44(7): 1025–36.

201. Crowell, D.T., et al. Weight change in the postpartum period. A review of the literature. *J Nurse Midwifery* 1995; 40(5): 418–23.

202. Quellec, A. L., et al. Weight loss in the post-partum period. *Rev Med Interne* 1995; 16(2): 251–3s.

203. Mosedale, L. Miscarriage: The Silent Loss. *Child* 1993; 85–95.

204. Stack, J. M., et al. The Psychodynamics of Spontaneous abortion. *American Journal of the Orthopsychiatric Association* 1984; 62.

205. Stay-Pederson, B., et al. Recurrent abortion: the role of psychotherapy in early pregnancy loss—mechanisms and treatment. London, England: *The Research Press*, 1988: pp. 433–40.

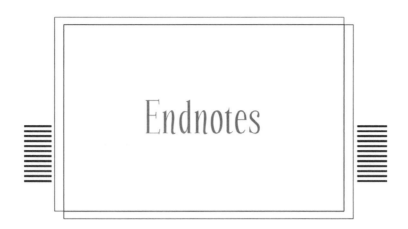

Endnotes

a) Groundbreaking research by the University of Surrey in the UK proves this. The research looked at 367 couples who were trying to conceive over a period of three years. The women were aged 22–45 and the men 25–59. Four out of ten had a history of infertility, and the same number had suffered repeated miscarriages. Many, especially those in the older age range, came to the pre-conception trial as a last resort. Over the past 25 years, the British organization Foresight has pioneered an approach to human fertility that takes into account diet, exposure to pollutants, infections, and nutritional status. The couples were instructed to follow a Foresight regime that involves detoxing, being tested for mineral and vitamin deficiencies and having these put right with supplements, and eating organic food. Any infections were treated. By the end of the trial, 90 percent of these couples had given birth to healthy babies. Even 65 percent of those who had tried IVF without success became pregnant naturally.

b) Data was drawn from a large 2002 multinational study—the European Study of Daily Fecundability. It enrolled 782 women aged 18–40 from seven centers: Milan, Verona, Lugano, Dusseldorf, Paris, London, and Brussels. The participants kept daily records of basal body temperature and recorded the days on which intercourse and menstrual bleeding occurred. Data on 7,288 menstrual cycles contributed to the study. Among outwardly healthy couples who failed to conceive naturally within the first year, many did conceive naturally in the second year, regardless of age. Research leader Dr. David Dunson recommends delaying assisted reproduction until a couple has failed to conceive naturally in 18–24 months, as this would avoid some of the well documented side effects associated with fertility treatments, such as miscarriage and low birth-weight.

c) At the University of Arkansas, 212 college students completed a survey designed to elicit information about their exercise habits, perceived sexual desirability, and body image. A number of body-image items were associated with both perceived physical attractiveness and perceived sexual desirability. Total body image was related to gender, exercise level, perceived physical attractiveness, perceived sexual desirability, and perception of self as a sexual partner.

d) Institute of Public Health, Department of Epidemiology, University of Southern Denmark, Denmark: They performed a study where they looked at the association between cigarette, alcohol, and caffeine consumption and the occurrence of spontaneous abortion. The conclusions were that consumption of five or more units of alcohol per week and 375 mg or more caffeine per day during pregnancy may increase the risk of spontaneous abortion. (See **v.rasch@dadlnet.dk** for more details.)

e) *New England Journal of Medicine:* One of the first large-scale studies found that even one day after ovulation the chance of getting pregnant drops dramatically. At the same time, researchers from the National Institute of Environmental Health Sciences in Research Park, North Carolina, also discovered that to ensure conception, the best time to begin making love is five days prior to ovulation as well as the day of ovulation itself. (1999)

f) In one study of female infertility, 53 patients with luteal phase defect (LPD) were treated with different Chinese medicinal herbs at different phases of their menstrual cycle. The patients were treated for three menstrual cycles; there was significant improvement in the luteal phase of endometrium, and a tendency for normalization of the wave forms and their amplitude after the treatment. The findings suggested that Chinese herbal medicines capable of replenishing the kidney could regulate the hypothalamus-pituitary-ovarian axis and thus improve the luteal function. Among the 53 cases, 22 (41.5%) conceived, but 68.18% of them required other measures to preserve the pregnancy.

g) Dubai London Clinic, UAE: The objective of this study was to assess the frequency of alternative medical usage in an prenatal population. A survey of alternative medicine usage was carried out among 305 consecutive patients over two months at their registration in mid-pregnancy at an Australian prenatal clinic. The study showed that something like 40 percent of patients used alternative medical therapy, 12 percent of which also used herbal therapy. No specific study of pregnancy outcome was carried out, but it is of concern that some herbs taken had the potential to adversely affect pregnancy outcome. The herbal therapies commonly used in pregnancy are reviewed with their potential complications; examples of toxicity are also discussed. It's important to obtain an herbal-medicine history at any time, but particularly in pregnancy. Herbs may have unrecognized effects on pregnancy or labor, have interactions with prescribed medications, and have potentially serious complications for the fetus.

h) Conclusions: Metformin therapy during pregnancy in women with PCOS was safely associated with reduction in SAB and in GD, wasn't teratogenic, and didn't adversely affect birth weight or height; or height, weight, and motor and social development at three and six months of age.

i) The trend for elective cesareans has been made popular by celebrities, but doctors point out that babies born by C-section are seven times more likely to suffer from breathing problems. While serious complications are rare, they can include hemorrhaging, scarring, and damage to the ovaries. It's also important to remember that a C-section is major surgery, and you'll need at least four weeks to recover, compared to a matter of days for women with natural births. Breast-feeding will be more difficult, and you'll need to stay in the hospital for longer. Around 60 percent of women who have a cesarean will still feel pain from the wound five months later.

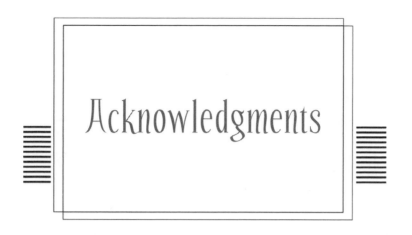

Acknowledgments

Colette:

A big thank-you to Theresa for being such a great, enthusiastic, and energetic colleague; to Hay House for being so supportive and helpful; to Chris for his steadfast support and kindness; to everyone at Verity and in the international PCOS community for their hard work getting PCOS on the map; to all the women who have contacted Theresa and me to share their stories and thoughts on dealing with PCOS—we couldn't have done it without you.

Theresa:

Thank you to Colette for being such an inspiration and joy to work with. Thank you to our editor, Michelle Pilley, for her support and encouragement. Thank you to Hay House. Thank you to Ray, and to my two beautiful children, Robert and Ruth, for their patience and love while I completed this project. Thank you to the many women with PCOS whom I spoke to in the course of writing this book. I am truly grateful for the insight you gave me.

Colette and Theresa:

Thank you to all the experts and advisors listed below for giving their time and thoughts to the questions asked, and sharing their knowledge with us and/or their important research on PCOS and fertility.

Dr. Adam Balen: consultant obstetrician and gynecologist and subspecialist in reproductive medicine and surgery, Leeds General Infirmary

Lucy Broughton: health journalist

Oscar Umahro Cadogan: lecturer at the Danish Institute of Optimal Nutrition

Dr. Adam Carey: London Nutritional Research Center

Dr. Gerard Conway: consultant gynecologist, Middlesex Hospital, London

Dr. Alice Domar: Harvard Medical School, Mind/Body research program

Dr. James Douglas: reproductive endocrinologist, Plano Medical Center, Plano, Texas

Dr. Robert Franklin: clinical professor of obstetrics and gynecology, Baylor College of Medicine, Houston, Texas.

Prof. Stephen Franks: professor of reproductive endocrinology, Imperial College, London

Jacqui Garnier, M.A.R.: reflexologist

Dr. Marilyn Glenville: nutritional therapist

Prof. Gabor Kovacs: director of obstetrics and gynecology, Monash University, Melbourne, Australia

Dr. Niels Lauersen: Obstetrician and gynecologist, St. Vincent Medical Center, New York

Dr. Helen Mason: senior lecturer in reproductive endocrinology, St. George's Hospital Medical School, London

Dr. Gillian McKeith: international nutritionist

Dr. Samuel Thatcher: expert in reproductive endocrinology serving on the advisory board of the American Infertility Association

Dr. Ann Walker: medical herbalist and nutrition research scientist, University of Reading

Toni Weschler: fertility awareness counseling and training seminars

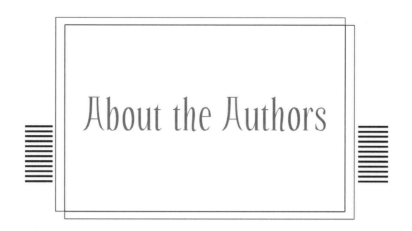

About the Authors

Colette Harris is a leading health journalist and magazine editor from the United Kingdom (U.K.) who was diagnosed with PCOS in 1996 and is currently wondering: *Will I be fertile if I decide I want children?* She has a degree from Oxford University and has been writing pioneering articles on PCOS in international newspapers and magazines since 1997 in order to raise awareness of the condition, and to campaign for better treatment and understanding for women who have it. Her passion is finding practical self-help strategies from nutrition to stress relief that have a profound effect on PCOS symptoms but also empower the women who use them. Colette is a frequent speaker at international conferences and women's groups exploring PCOS.

Theresa Cheung is a freelance writer, teacher, health consultant, and mom who was diagnosed with PCOS in 1997 when she was trying to conceive. At that time, Theresa was living in the U.S., where she had her first child using fertility drugs, and she then completed her family with fertility treatment in the U.K. Theresa holds a master's degree from Cambridge University and now divides her time between the U.S. and the U.K.

Colette and Theresa have used their personal experiences and expertise to publish their previous books, *The PCOS Diet Book* and *You Can Beat PMS*.

We hope you enjoyed this Hay House book.
If you'd like to receive a free catalog featuring additional
Hay House books and products, or if you'd like information about
the Hay Foundation, please contact:

Hay House, Inc.
P.O. Box 5100
Carlsbad, CA 92018-5100

(760) 431-7695 or **(800) 654-5126**
(760) 431-6948 (fax) or **(800) 650-5115 (fax)**
www.hayhouse.com®

———

Published and distributed in Australia by:
Hay House Australia Pty. Ltd., 18/36 Ralph St., Alexandria NSW 2015
Phone: 612-9669-4299 • *Fax:* 612-9669-4144 • www.hayhouse.com.au

Published and distributed in the United Kingdom by:
Hay House UK, Ltd., 292B Kensal Rd., London W10 5BE • *Phone:*
44-20-8962-1230 • *Fax:* 44-20-8962-1239 • www.hayhouse.co.uk

Published and distributed in the Republic of South Africa by:
Hay House SA (Pty), Ltd., P.O. Box 990, Witkoppen 2068 • *Phone/Fax:*
27-11-467-8904 • orders@psdprom.co.za • www.hayhouse.co.za

Published in India by: Hay House Publishers India,
Muskaan Complex, Plot No. 3, B-2, Vasant Kunj, New Delhi 110 070
Phone: 91-11-4176-1620 • *Fax:* 91-11-4176-1630 • www.hayhouse.co.in

Distributed in Canada by: Raincoast, 9050 Shaughnessy St.,
Vancouver, B.C. V6P 6E5 • *Phone:* (604) 323-7100
Fax: (604) 323-2600 • www.raincoast.com

———

Tune in to **HayHouseRadio.com®** for the best in
inspirational talk radio featuring top Hay House authors!
And, sign up via the Hay House USA Website to receive the Hay House
online newsletter and stay informed about what's going on with your
favorite authors. You'll receive bimonthly announcements about
Discounts and Offers, Special Events, Product Highlights, Free Excerpts,
Giveaways, and more!
www.hayhouse.com®